Electra vs Oedipus

Electra vs Oedipus explores the deeply complex and often turbulent relationship between mothers and daughters. In contrast to Sigmund Freud's conviction that the father is the central figure, the book puts forward the notion that women are in fact far more (pre)occupied with their mother.

Drawing on the author's extensive clinical experience, the book provides numerous case studies that shed light on women's emotional development. Topics include:

- love and hate between mothers and daughters
- the history of maternal love
- childbirth and depression
- rejected mothers.

Electra vs Oedipus will be a valuable resource for psychoanalysts, psychotherapists, and all those with an interest in the dynamics of the mother–daughter relationship.

Hendrika C. Freud is a Psychoanalyst and a Member of The International Psychoanalytic Association and Association for Child Psychoanalysis. She is a teacher, supervisor, and training analyst of the Dutch Psychoanalytic Society and The Dutch Psychoanalytic Association and has been in private practice for nearly fifty years.

Electra vs Oedipus

The drama of the mother–daughter relationship

Hendrika C. Freud

Translated from the Dutch by
Marjolijn de Jager

The translation for this edition was made possible
with financial support from the Dutch Foundation
for Literature

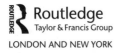

Routledge
Taylor & Francis Group

LONDON AND NEW YORK

First published in Amsterdam in 1997
by Uitgeverji Van Gennep BV as
Electra versus Oedipus, Psychoanalytische Visies op de Moeder-Dochter Relatie

First published in the UK in 2011
by Routledge
27 Church Road, Hove, East Sussex BN3 2FA

Simultaneously published in the USA and Canada
by Routledge
711 Third Avenue, New York, NY 10017

*Routledge is an imprint of the Taylor & Francis Group,
an Informa business*

© C Van Gennep Amsterdam
Translation © 2010 Marjolijn de Jager

The right of Hendrika C. Freud to be identified as author of this
work has been asserted by her in accordance with sections
77 and 78 of the Copyright, Designs and Patents Act 1988.

Typeset in Times by
RefineCatch Limited, Bungay, Suffolk
Printed and bound in Great Britain by
TJ International Ltd, Padstow, Cornwall
Paperback cover design by Andrew Ward

This publication has been produced with paper manufactured to
strict environmental standards and with pulp derived from
sustainable forests.

British Library Cataloguing in Publication Data
A catalogue record for this book is available from the British Library

Library of Congress Cataloging-in-Publication Data
Halberstadt-Freud, Hendrika C., 1937–
  [Electra versus Oedipus. English]
  Electra vs Oedipus : the drama of the mother–daughter
  relationship / Hendrika C. Freud.
    p. cm.
  1. Electra complex. I. Title.
  BF175.5.E45H3513 2010
  155.6′463—dc22   2010005928

ISBN: 978-0-415-54796-3 (hbk)
ISBN: 978-0-415-54797-0 (pbk)

For my daughter,
Jutka Halberstadt

Contents

Preface

This is a book about women, and I hope that it will lead to a better understanding of the relationship between mothers and daughters. As a psychoanalyst, over nearly fifty years I have spoken with many mothers and many daughters. It became increasingly more obvious to me that a re-orientation towards female development was inevitable. The result of my reflections is *Electra vs Oedipus: The Drama of the Mother–Daughter Relationship*.

I have described the distorted relationships that men are capable of having with their mothers in the book *Freud, Proust, Perversion and Love* (1991). Over the course of time it has struck me that actually women become entangled far more frequently with their mothers.

These distorted mother–daughter relationships led me to reflect upon existing psychoanalytic theories and the flaws they contained. The Oedipus complex, as it had been dealt with and popularized for more than a century, cannot automatically be applied to the woman. This old model argues that a little boy is in love with his mother, a little girl with her father, and that later on each of them will look for someone else able to actualize the continuation of this romance. According to this view, a woman searches for a man who resembles her father because as a little girl she was already in love with this first hero in her life.

However, it turns out to be more complicated than that. For boys the mother is the first person they encounter in this world, with all the fateful results thereof. What is all too often forgotten is that the same thing holds true for girls – for them, too, love relationships go back to their first love object, and that is the mother, not the father. (Subject and object are psychoanalytic terms that refer to the two individuals in a relationship.)

The past thirty years have produced much greater clarity in the vicissitudes of female development. Nevertheless, the Oedipus myth continued to be valid for men as well as women. Partly because of this, the secret of the woman remained a dark continent to which only a few were able to gain access.

The time has come to adapt the fundamental myth of psychoanalysis and expand it to make it more applicable to women. It is my hope that this book will contribute to this effort.

I would like to express my gratitude to my patients for the confidence they have had in me and for all that I have learned thanks to them. The names in the case descriptions have been changed, as have some of the characteristics, in order to ensure anonymity.

Chapter 1

Love and hate between mothers and daughters

The character of Electra dates back to ancient Greek mythology. Various playwrights, such as Aeschylus, Sophocles, and Euripides, devoted tragedies to her, and, for the latter in particular, mother and daughter are at the heart of the play. Everything that could possibly go wrong between the two of them is described in these works.

It is not without reason that, through the centuries, even after the classical era, Electra has continued to be an inspiration for many authors. The legendary Electra was far more preoccupied with her mother, whom she hated, than with the father she adored. Agamemnon, her father, had left home ten years before the setting of the play, when he departed for Troy as military commander to fight for the liberation of the beautiful Helen who had been abducted – thereby triggering or actually causing the Trojan War. In the meantime, Electra's mother Clytemnestra had taken a new lover. Electra feels neglected and rejected by her. She is jealous of her mother but also of her mother's lover. Excluded from all intimacy, she wanders around the palace, moaning and cursing.

Electra dislikes her role as a woman. She rebuffs all thoughts of sexuality. She has no desire to marry, and, if that does have to happen, she certainly wants no children. Her histrionic personality inspires loathing from every corner. Electra has become the prototype of a woman with female problems.

She is a domineering victim who manages to conceal her insecurity and yearning for motherly love beneath a great deal of noise. She disparages her more feminine sister and uses her brother Orestes as a tool to avenge herself on her mother. Taking revenge on this detested mother is her only goal in life. Her youth, her beauty – she sacrifices them all for this one purpose. After many bitter and sorrowful years, filled with pain, she succeeds in her scheme: her mother is murdered as she pleads for mercy.

This is a brief outline of the image we see when we look at Electra from the outside. But how does Electra herself experience her dilemmas, what is her psychic reality, what are her unconscious conflicts?

Briefly told and magnified as only possible in a work of art, the mythical Electra figure shows many of the unconscious preoccupations with which women with problems may be struggling. For instance, the fear of being swallowed up by the powerful mother figure is in conflict with a desperate longing for her love and affection. But masochistic complaints, depression, and sexual inhibitions are frequently manifested as well. All of them are problems that relate back to the very first love object, the mother – just as with Electra.

Culture has changed and is changeable, but certain situations are set in stone. Girls begin their life in a homosexual love relationship – in the sense of with a person of the same sex – with a woman: their mother. Not until later is the heterosexual love for their father added.

Paradoxical as that may sound, girls need their mother's cooperation in detaching themselves from her. Sometimes that opportunity for independence is lacking, and women have to find a way to sail between the Scylla of Electra's murderous hate and the Charybdis of total symbiosis. Both extremes lead to an unhealthy mother–daughter relationship. As always, it is only the happy medium that can progress to a healthy development.

The father is often idealized and, just as Electra's father, he is missed or lamented in his absence. Often fathers are absent or too little involved with their children, who therefore have to rely on their mother. The girl attempts to direct herself to her father when he is available. If not, she must make do with her fantasies. Sometimes she has a chance to receive the love for which she yearns from her father, the love that she may not have been given by her mother. Sometimes that attempt fails. A second disappointment is then the sad result. However, even if it does succeed, her mother remains the primary object of her desire, which is at best transferred to her father.

Subsequently, for a healthy development it is necessary for the image of the omnipotent mother, the goddess, or the queen of childhood fantasy to be abandoned. In psychoanalytic theory this figure is known as the phallic mother, because she is simultaneously both man and woman, as it were. After all, for small children the difference between the sexes is not very clear yet. The fantasy that an individual can be both man and woman is discarded with some difficulty. Even with regard to themselves, girls and women often continue to struggle with their bisexual identity.

The Electra complex is meant not to replace the Oedipus complex but to complement it.[1] The new discoveries around the cliffs that the woman must steer clear of in her development are, in my opinion, better suited to a model in which it is not the father but the mother who occupies centre stage.

Symbiosis, meaning the mutual dependency of two beings, is problematic if taken as a phase of development. Mother and child do, of course, have idyllic moments when they are completely wrapped up in each other. But when a mother feels constantly dependent on her child's endorsement, there is a disorder at play. This can express itself, for example, in the need for a child to cling to its mother when she is leaving because she would otherwise have the sense that she is not a good mother. I call this unhealthy mutual dependency the *symbiotic illusion*. It is a disorder that impedes the normal maturation process. When such a bond between mother and daughter remains intact for life, there is not enough room for independence and other relationships.

The opposite of the *symbiotic illusion* – namely, total separation – is equally inauspicious. Under ideal circumstances the girl partially detaches herself from the mother. A girl needs to be able to shape her own identity but, at the same time, continues to need her mother throughout her life as model and counsellor.

Due to the open borders between mothers and daughters, styles of mothering and motherhood are transmitted from generation to generation. This can be fortunate or harmful. Transgenerational transmission of traumas is a well-known phenomenon and, obviously, not only along the female line, although it is especially visible, forceful, and inescapable there.

For a woman, the inner bond with the mother can be a source both of strength and of frustration. To a great extent, the child's first relationship is decisive for its identity and sense of self-worth, particularly among women. Subsequent love relationships can be damaged when a woman continues to see herself as the extension of her mother. Then mother and daughter keep mirroring themselves in each other, as in the fairy tale of Snow White: 'Mirror, mirror on the wall, who is the loveliest of them all?' Involuntarily, such a daughter remains inside her mother's range of influence and will continue to be a part of her mother, body and soul. Instead of her own desires, she must fulfil her mother's wishes. The instinctive result of this is hostility towards her mother, often hidden even from herself.

The way in which unconscious feelings of hatred can colour and decide the emotional life of a daughter is the principal theme of this book. Separation is related to autonomy. Women often interpret their detachment as a form of aggression that might harm the mother. Thus they tend to conceal their anger and turn it against themselves in the form of headaches, feelings of guilt, or masochism. The purpose of this book is to use the fateful struggle of Electra as a paradigm for conflicts in female development.

We shall see that the Oedipus paradigm in girls frequently ends in an Electra complex – that is to say: rage with the mother and idealization of the father. The other extreme, the 'symbiotic illusion' with the mother, appears frequently as well. This prevents the girl from growing into an independent person. Consequently, she is basically unable to enter into an adult heterosexual relationship. In her intimate relationships she will tend to claim the other, to cling to or fuse with that person. The symbiotic illusion as quasi-intimacy makes the other invisible as a separate individual.

A sound theory is indispensable in confronting reality, but everyday practice is still the most fascinating. Recently, Tessa, a beautiful and well-educated young woman, came into my consultation room with a mysteriously amused look on her face. This shy woman with a soft voice smiled at me with a mixture of 'glad to see you', with alarm in her gaze, and with unambiguous triumph, almost a note of pity. When questioned, she burst into uncontrollable laughter that at the same time she was ashamed of, as if she were betraying something about herself that would have been better left concealed. Then an elaborate panorama unfolded around her and her parents, who had divorced early on.

Tessa's mother had trouble listening to and being interested in her, while her father, a childlike and egocentric man who was more seductive than interested, always praised her to the sky to others. This habitually led to scenes that were embarrassing to her, whereby she was pushed forward as her father's showpiece. A contrasting scenario was played out with her mother. Being small and helpless without a trace of hostility produced at least a bit of attention in this distant and overburdened mother. Stepping more into the limelight would only have elicited rejection, Tessa feared.

Upon closer examination it turned out that Tessa had always been afraid of her mother's jealousy. She was quite astonished when I first articulated that possibility. Her mother, who had not had much education, never quite knew what her daughter was studying. During therapy it became clear quite quickly what a taboo existed for her in competing with me as a woman. This ambitious, highly competitive young woman had learned to live with a hidden identity. She was terrified of the murderous envy that in her fantasy she might incite if she were to be successful, and she had therefore learned to conceal her triumphs beneath a great show of modesty.

This example illustrates how the Oedipus story about patricide and the little boy's love for the mother is not automatically applicable to a girl.[2] Of course, there is a vital attraction between the sexes and being different continues to be the most exciting thing there is. But the gratification of a girl's desires often has a great deal more to do with her mother than with her father.

Chapter 2

The symbiotic illusion

In families of today the mother is the most influential person and is therefore held responsible for everything that might go wrong in the rearing of the child. Because ideal mothers are just as rare as model children, the two can easily become disappointed with each other.

Mothers may pay too little or too much attention, and as a result children may feel neglected or burdened. However, parenthood does not consist merely of conscious interaction with children. Even more important are the messages that are unconsciously transmitted. Moreover, the 'repetition compulsion' – patterns repeating themselves in successive generations – plays a large role as well. A mother who is disappointed in her own mother will be more than likely to have an unusually ambivalent relationship with her daughter. An anxious mother will be less able to keep the fears of her child within bounds.

Depending on the experiences in their own childhood, parents will reflect or distort reality and have a coloured view of that reality. In that sense, grandparents may be rediscovered as an important influence two generations later. Many experiences of the parents are projected automatically onto the next generation, on the children. A father who feels rejected by his father may have a tendency to reject his son, even if only occasionally, or – vice versa – may feel rejected by his son. The stamp that parents imprint on the child will induce similar patterns in subsequent generations. This is particularly true when a family endured experiences that are traumatic in nature. As the Russian novelist Leo Tolstoy expressed it in *Anna Karenina*: 'All happy families are alike, but every unhappy family is unhappy in its own way.'

Aïda

Aïda is a vastly overweight student who suffers from severe headaches and always feels on edge. She explains that her mother calls her every day and always wants to see her more than once a week. They then have long discussions about how to live, a topic on which her mother has all kinds of theories and ideas. During these conversations Aïda asks for advice and help with her problems. This way she provokes her mother to give advice that she can reject in an adolescent way, thereby staying over-involved.

Aïda tries to build a similar relationship with me as her therapist. She always sits on the edge of her chair, cannot relax for a minute, and constantly picks at her lips. At the same time she tries to provoke a discussion in response to every remark I make. She impresses me as someone who is in need of excessive interaction: something has to keep flying back and forth between us, as if she cannot be left to her own devices for a second when she is around me. I have to offer my opinion on everything, and when I occasionally do so, I have to prove that I am right – and so on, ad infinitum.

Any time I say anything, Aïda interrupts with a 'but'. This is followed by an argument that expresses doubt about what I had just said, which in turn is followed by a plea to remove her doubts. Or else she starts to argue for the opposite to my suggestion. It produces a sense that nothing is ever right, is ever sufficient, and that there is never room for a pause or a moment of contentment. Everything continues to be one long line of pure frustration. It is as if she can never be fully satisfied.

Her role within the family was, and still is, that of meeting the needs of the others. She was always the obedient daughter who, in contrast to her three brothers, never caused her parents any problems. In addition, Aïda has always taken care of her paternal grandmother as well. Her studies are going well, while her brothers are neither working nor studying – they are living on welfare with their wives and children. Rather than independence and self-reliance, dependency seems to be the life theme of the children in this family. If Aïda is not constantly in touch with her mother, she feels guilty, just like her mother, who always feels she is remiss in her duties towards her daughter. Neither of them is able to loosen the reins and let the other be.

Aïda's father had been in hiding during the Second World War, and he had lost his own father at an early age. Her grandfather was killed in Auschwitz, making her a second-generation victim of war trauma. Her father was raised by his mother and grandmother. His mother is a true survivor, who leans heavily on Aïda while urging her on to ever greater accomplishments. Aïda feels responsible for this grandmother, who is by now very old and rather difficult, especially because her own parents do not want to bother with her too much and leave most of the care to Aïda.

Aïda's father keeps a safe distance from the family by burying himself in his work. He has married a woman who tries to patch up her own unhappy childhood by overprotecting her husband and children. However, only with Aïda does she completely succeed in this. She wants to know everything about her daughter and to meddle in all her affairs. Aïda involuntarily fuels this attitude. These two, mother and daughter, behave as if they were married to one another instead of to their male partners. The symbiotic illusion that binds them is detrimental to Aïda's development as an independent woman and creates problems that contribute to her compulsive brooding and to the headaches from which she suffers.

Emma

Another example is Emma, a woman in her fifties, widowed, with two children, and now happily remarried. Her children are grown and she lives an extremely comfortable life, and yet she complains that she cannot find any peace. She has to achieve, study, work, travel. She has to improve herself constantly, worry whether she is handling her children, her stepchildren, and her husband properly. She is tired and wants to be rid of this attitude to life but is unable to let go of it all.

At the age of 3 Emma had lost her mother and was raised by a detached father and a hostile stepmother, both of them extremely demanding strict Calvinists. At least, that is how Emma experienced it. She escaped from the parental home when she was 18, went to work, married, and had children. However, she soon had the feeling that she and her husband were not well matched. She felt as if she was imprisoned in a cage, she seemed to be suffocating. She was never able to show any true emotions to her husband, so that sexuality became problematic as well. Her husband had become the replacement for her cold and distant stepmother. She never realized that it might all have to do with the lack of a loving mother – a lack from which she had suffered deeply.

During one summer vacation Emma suddenly fell madly in love with another man who, according to her, was the love of her life. Coincidentally or not, her husband became severely depressed soon thereafter and committed suicide. Emma felt incredibly guilty and ashamed, a feeling that has remained until today. Not long afterwards her secret friend died as well. For the second time she lost the most beloved person in her life.

In her own eyes, Emma's first husband resembled her stepmother, while the bond she had with her lover was more of a representation of the primal emotion she must at one time have had with her mother. Her present husband is a survivor of World War II, and, as happens quite often in marriages, through a mechanism called projective identification, his losses come to represent her own loss of a mother. Being with him, she experiences what she has never dared to admit to herself – that she has always missed her mother enormously. This way she can identify with her husband and need not dwell on the great loss in her life.

What struck me most in Emma was that she never really emphasized the fact that her mother had died so young. Her grief about that was so much a part of her prehistory that she was incapable of dealing with it until we were able to bring it to light during her treatment sessions. I surmised that the main cause of her discomfort was to be found in this, her unprocessed sorrow. She had spent her entire childhood among strangers, as it were, without any sense of intimacy. With me, by contrast, she felt at ease with remarkable and surprising speed. After a few sessions she began to weep, saying that she was deeply moved by her visits to me although she did not quite understand why. In fact, though she was always trying to be as distant and as rational as possible, I felt that she radiated great affection.

After we continued to work through her mourning and made connections with her current life, her emotions grew more recognizable to Emma, and she became calmer, less driven. It was no longer so urgent that she seek intense activity in the outside world just so she would not notice what was really going on inside her. I felt very strongly that via her transference to me in treatment she had retrieved an old emotion that originally belonged with her little-girl's feeling for her mother. That bond, which had been severed before she was old enough to be aware of what was happening, was found again in the present moment; the wish for symbiosis was thereby resolved, and she could leave me with a feeling of satisfaction.

In love with the therapist

The baby's first relationship is with the mother. This bond is very different for boys than it is for girls. Mothers have a tendency – an obviously very subtle one – to eroticize the bond with boys more, while with girls they actually try to curb that aspect. In part because of this, girls are generally more restrained sexually. In addition, they keep yearning for their first love object more than boys do. The unfulfilled symbiotic need of women can become a source of suffering and depression, and not infrequently this is what makes them seek out a psychotherapist.

In my experience, women have a tendency to fall in love with their female therapist, often without being aware of it. The idealizing symbiotic atmosphere of unspoken mutual understanding, of together being one, of solidarity through thick and thin, of admiration, is generated remarkably more often during the treatment of women than that of men. In my experience men may well fall in love with their female therapist and even make some clumsy attempts at seduction, but only so they will not have to talk about what they actually came for. Women, on the other hand, are often not at all aware of how strongly they express their – usually not sexually tinged – feelings of being in love to their female therapist. It is as if in the therapeutic situation they fall in love in a very different and special way – that is to say, as if they have found their first love object, their mother, again, or the mother they never had, the mother who did not love them or loved them insufficiently, the one for whom they had always longed. In the transference relationship, women often have idyllic unconscious fantasies around their female therapist.

Most women manage to transfer the love for their mother only partially to a man. After all, love for the father was added quite early on to the love for the mother. Even women who have passed through these stages and are crazy about their father, and later their husband, often still foster a secret, deeply concealed wish for a loving mother.

Men have to suppress their desire to be dependent and are able to satisfy it later on. Many a man can find maternal care with his beloved, and the contact with this wife or female partner can often be more satisfying than it ever was with the mother.

Women, on the other hand, seem less capable of finding complete satisfaction in a man, whether that relationship is successful or not. They continue to nurture a nameless longing for the affection of women and find that in friendships with women.

Mary

The example of Mary illustrates that the symbiotic yearnings for motherly love can conceal much hate. She came to see me because of depression following the birth of her first child. To her great anger and grief, her hypochondriac mother had died just before Mary delivered her baby. Moreover, throughout her childhood and youth she had been heavily burdened by the fact that she has a severely handicapped younger sister.

Her mother suffered from all sorts of ailments, imaginary or not, and was often in bed, either at home or in hospital. She would then constantly call on her daughter, who had to be present, had to pay attention, could never wander far from home, and was not allowed to do anything without first discussing it extensively with her mother. Mary was crazy about her father, a peaceful man who did not say much but did not intervene either when mother and daughter went too far in their mutual clinging. Whenever her father did take her side, Mary would feel guilty towards her mother.

The postnatal depression followed much more longstanding problems but expressed itself only after the birth of her first child. Mary cried a lot and was desperately unhappy because, in her own eyes, she was never good or good enough in what she did. She had always been trying to accommodate everyone else, and that was not getting any better at this point. Because she was unable to say 'no' to anyone at work either, she became utterly exhausted.

Mary had the feeling that her mother had abandoned her at the very moment she needed her most, and she missed her continually. At the same time, she gradually began to realize that her mother had never been able to give her any support but actually had relied more on her. The warm symbiotic relationship she thought she remembered and for which she so yearned turned out to have been more of an excessive mutual claiming. She had never been aware that she was angry with her mother: she had always repressed her irritation in order to experience the quasi-intimate atmosphere they both loved so much.

To be sure, mother and daughter chatted much and often, but their conversation was inane and innocuous, although Mary is an intelligent woman.

They did not exchange anything personal or confidential. Expressing what she thought of her mother, not to mention any kind of criticism, was strictly taboo. Mary was often bored in her mother's presence and felt empty and disgruntled. She had the sense of being locked up with her well-intentioned parents, which, in turn, made her feel guilty towards them.

The unexpressed mutual contract with her mother consisted of the obligation to be as helpful to each other as possible, even if it was at the expense of Mary's freedom. When she had still lived at home, her mother would always wait up for her until she came in at night. Although Mary did not want her to, her mother stayed up, no matter what the hour. Then Mary would feel guilty, but this was never discussed openly: there was always an implicit reproach in the air. Mary tried to meet her mother halfway in everything, no matter how constrained she felt. She never detached herself from her mother and always continued to be the dependent, affectionate child.

'I could have just killed her, and yet I can't do without her', Mary says about her dead mother. 'When she was still alive, I was always trying to keep her at a distance, and at the same time I always longed for her.' The same pattern is repeated with her little daughter, who can be extremely coercive. It infuriates her that the child elicits the very thing in her that so bothered her in her mother. Yet, she tries to satisfy every one of her little girl's whims. The child is afraid of witches; that seems to be where she projects the aggression between mother and child that is not to be noticed.

Women like Mary feel lonely and abandoned when there is no one on their back. When a relationship is not parasitic, it means you do not love each other. Thinking the same thoughts, feeling the same feelings, resembling each other, and wanting the same things are all part of the deceptive world of the symbiotic illusion – deceptive because, upon closer consideration, the stronger the symbiosis, the less two people have in common. A clinging intimacy is simply quite different from a true exchange of real empathy and interest in the other person. It is never self-evident, and it is actually rare for two people to have the same thoughts and feelings, as the symbiotic illusion supposes. Mary finds it necessary that the other is constantly on the same wavelength. In everything she does, she seeks my approval. She is always afraid that I might disapprove of her. She feels that she must adopt the attitude of being small and dependent in order to acquire the approval of women who remind her of her mother.

A closer look at symbiosis

What I call the symbiotic illusion is the mutual psychological involvement that leads to extreme interdependence. It refers to the inseparability of the mother inside the head of the daughter, and vice versa. 'When I think of my mother, I am one with her.' The illusion of being one together is shared by both parties, each from her own perspective. This symbiotic illusion obstructs further development, for which at least some measure of autonomy, separation, or individuation is needed. Far from being limited to parent and child, the illusion can be encountered at any age as an inner interaction scenario.

For a long time symbiosis had been seen as a normal stage in the early development of the child. But symbiosis is a term that refers more to idealization than to the reality.[1] The idyll of the mother with the little child as a sacred duality is deceptive.

Mother and child are, of course, very intimately connected for a while, and there certainly are blissful moments of duality to be seen. But in the end the mother is still her own person and not dependent upon the child in the way that the child is on her. If all is well, the mother has a life of her own apart from her child, she has a love relationship with her husband or partner from which the child is excluded, and there is no mutual dependency, as is the case in an unhealthy development.

Some children, like Emma, miss a close connection with a mother because she disappeared from their lives too soon. Other mothers feel no need for physical contact or tenderness and remain aloof from their child. Obviously, neither of these two extremes is ideal. The third unhealthy possibility is total symbiosis. When the mother leans on her child emotionally, when the child is the centre of her attention to the exclusion of all other interests, when all satisfaction in her life depends on her child, this will hamper its development.

For the pact with the devil that is thus created, I have come up with the term symbiotic illusion, as mentioned above. It is a matter of a dyad, a duo chained and addicted to each other, out of a feeling of guilt more than of love, and the signs of affection are never sufficient or satisfying. It is an oppressive interaction that occurs more frequently in mothers and daughters than in mothers and sons. In the latter case the results are more conspicuous, as we shall see in a number of examples later in this chapter.

The symbiotic illusion is a matter of the mother providing the child with love on condition that he or she surrender to her wishes. That the mother's equilibrium depends on her satellite remains hidden. The child, even when adult, must continue to give signs of how impossible it is to do without the mother, thus reassuring her and giving her the feeling that she is indispensable and a good mother. The symbiotic illusion is a strongly narcissistic bond that serves to keep the mother's vulnerable sense of self-worth intact as much as possible. The fact is that a child does not like to feel that it cannot rely on a rock-solid mother. Children are extraordinarily sensitive to the weaknesses, doubts, and uncertainties in their mothers. Weak mothers can be experienced as being extremely peremptory, in the way that only helplessness, illness, or vulnerability can be peremptory.

The duality of the symbiosis is expressed through the exclusion of a third party, on whom all hostility might be projected. While excessive identification with one parent – usually the mother – is taking place, the other is kept out. Thus the symbiotic alliance hinders triangulation, another word for the oedipal or triangular relationship between parents and child. Furthermore, separation and individuation are thereby also rendered more difficult.

The child's sense of self, its sense of self-worth, is reduced because of an excessive dependency from which a sense of failure ensues. On the other hand, the child often feels a position of independence, a detaching from the mother, as too aggressive. Women in particular suffer from this. When a girl detaches herself from her mother, she fears that it might hurt her or, worse, be a direct attack on a mother who is too weak to handle it. When the girl goes her own way, it disturbs the balance of the indispensable symbiotic duality. Many women have a tendency to solve their conflicts masochistically by directing hostility and aggression towards themselves. Anger or rebellion does not belong in the idyllic love relationship of the symbiotic couple.

All too often psychological complaints have to do with this relationship model. Mother and child are so chained to one another that no mortal can come between them. Clinging to each other firmly will prevent the possibility of attacking each other, it impedes rivalry – in short, it is one way of avoiding aggression, an unhealthy situation that may develop during babyhood and dominate later life. It is less a question here of a real than of an internalized mother – that is to say, the mother is inside the child's head, even if she is long dead, as was the case with Mary.

When the father is emotionally or physically absent and will not or cannot intervene to break through a mother–daughter bond that is too intense, when in the mother's experience he plays no role as her child's father, when the mother seeks her fulfilment in the child, the mother–child dyad will not become a triad. The oedipal phase or triangulation, wherein the child must recognize that it is not alone in the world with its mother, will be achieved inadequately or not at all. We see a repetition of the above-mentioned relationship model in the transference. A semblance of harmony with the therapist is kept up without any overt aggression. Hidden anger and fear will then lead to dreams filled with blood and mayhem, or to violent fantasies that are thinly suppressed.

Although I originally thought I encountered the symbiotic illusion most clearly in male perversions and male homosexuality, it appears certainly not to be limited to such cases but is much more widely spread as a fundamental structure.[2] In psychosis, this state of affairs is often clearly recognizable, but its important influences are also to be found among the less pernicious disorders such as psychoneuroses, as well as among borderline patients.

The illusion is based on the idea: 'We love only each other, no one else in the world matters', which contains a false harmony. The contract that is implicitly made is an exchange along the lines of: 'As long as I endorse you as a perfect mother, you won't show that you hate me when I don't oblige you.' On the contrary: 'If I give you the feeling you're a good mother and obediently do what you expect and want from me, you might give me the expressions of love I need.' Independence exchanged for love is rewarded with seductive overindulgence and physical care.

The 'goodnight kiss episode' in *Remembrance of Things Past* by the French author Marcel Proust can serve as an illustration of this. The mother wants her son to be strong and manly, so she refuses the goodnight kiss, but later she gives in to his whims. She makes a pact with her son, from which the father is excluded. She subsequently gives in to her son's wishes on condition that he remain dependent. In Proust's earlier novel *Jean Santeuil*, in his short stories, as in *Remembrance of Things Past*, he illustrates how a homosexual and rather perverse youth attempts to salvage his independence from the excessive dependence on and identification with his mother. She counsels him against going out with his friends, 'He is better off doing his homework, not wasting his time. Going out and having fun will only make him ill, it's dangerous for him' – in short, he is much better off staying safely with his mother. He hides his anger, has secret relationships, and feels guilty.

Moreover, the protagonist or narrator is always asthmatic, just as Proust himself was. Being ill and dependent helps to seal the pact with his mother. She says, in effect: 'As long as you need me, I will be good to you. As soon as you leave me, I will hate you.' The child fears that hate and submissively keeps doing what the mother needs. The resulting indulgence goes hand in hand with clear neglect in the sense that the child is not seen as a separate person, with its own needs. He feels himself to be merely the extension of his mother. His private desires, detached from her, do not count. This pampering can easily lead to an almost incestuous intimacy. The relationship crosses all borders and forms a psychic assault that is no less serious than a physical one.

Several male examples follow here, because they reflect the situation of the symbiotic illusion in a less veiled form and they speak more clearly than is often the case with women. The syndromes in men are more bizarre because of the gender difference and the measures required to protect their male identity.

Ernest

Ernest is a gifted 40-year-old man, a physicist who struggles with serious social problems. He is homosexual and lives alone. He and his mother have always been extremely preoccupied with each other. Still, they had no real contact. In fact, they knew very little about each other's private thoughts and feelings. They never exchanged any personal information or real intimacy. She was simply always there to please him. He was her idol. After her death, he was incapable of feeling anything like grief. He does not even know whether he misses her.

This mother lost her brother when he was deported during the war; her trauma was never processed or verbalized, but the loss hung tangibly suspended in the air. Ernest sensed that he was meant to replace someone, had to be his mother's solace, had to support her in her unuttered sorrow. She would constantly send non-verbal messages that he had to decode. He tried to please her as much as possible. In exchange, he received her unconditional affection and approval. He mattered more than her husband, who always remained in the background.

Although there was not much warmth between mother and son, the hate that was undoubtedly there as well remained profoundly concealed. Deep into his treatment Ernest finally begins to wonder whether it had all been so perfect. He behaves as if his mother is still alive, although she has been dead for ten years. His symbiosis with her has never been resolved. He is still one with her. His internalized mother is his guardian angel who is always perched on his shoulder, and he is still her little boy. Sometimes he has the feeling that he is literally becoming his mother – for instance when he is a host and feels more like a hostess, doing everything the way his mother used to do.

During his analysis this symbiotic duality is completely transferred to me. We can never disagree for a minute, our bond is self-evident, he tries to please me and wants my unconditional presence and attention as a reward. When I go on holiday, there is a problem. My absence is denied. He forgets dates that have been set. He does weird things and has bizarre delusions during the interruptions in the treatment. It may vary from suffering fierce hypo-chondriac attacks, phoning the AIDS information line to ask whether he could have AIDS (without any sexual contact or having taken any risks, however), breaking a leg, selling his mother's furniture (as Marcel did in *Remembrance of Things Past* with the furniture of his Aunt Léonie), shaving his head, and so forth. The least aberrant thing that happens is that he falls in love with a rather unlikely partner.

The curious thing in all this is that Ernest never sees any connection between his antics and accidents during my absence and his emotional reaction to separation and abandonment. His denial works at the cost of reality. Mother is always there, and should she not be there, this would break their pact so painfully that it is entirely inconceivable. Ernest reacts to my absence by unconsciously cutting off all connections to me. That is his defence mechanism and survival strategy. He never misses anyone – he simply never feels that emotion.

The symbiotic illusion functions in a separate split-off part of consciousness. Hate and aggression have been tucked away in a separate part of the computer known as the mind. Normal reality exists as well, in the more conscious section. Ernest often lives in a cocoon: he sees others only to the extent that they can be of use to him, he is absorbed in his own fantasies. The idyll with the inner mother in which Ernest lives excludes not only any difference of opinion, but also any separation. The difference in gender and generation does not exist either: Ernest thinks that he and I are contemporaries, while in reality I am far older than he.

Peter

An example from the realm of perversions can further illustrate the symbiotic illusion because, just as in the dream, here an often caricatured scenario encompasses the manifestation of a yet-to-be-deciphered latent content. Peter has sought treatment because of marital problems and regularly occurring episodes of secret cross-dressing. In the course of his therapy he increasingly discovers that he is always concealing himself behind a mask and hiding from others. He is constantly pretending – his entire life is one continuous travesty of hiding his true self. He tries to imperceptibly manipulate his interlocutor and inveigle this person into validating him. It is necessary for him to always be in line with the other, while disagreement, not to mention overt protest or resistance, is impossible.

His contact consists exclusively of calculating how he can bring another person to say that he is right, that he is doing fine, and so on. He constantly wants to be praised or, at the very least, to be reassured. Time and again his wife is obliged to confirm that she loves him, ad nauseam, although he knows perfectly well that she has had enough of his questioning. He has a very close relationship with his mother. She still decides what is good for him and what clothes he and his children, too, should wear. Without being asked, she then makes those purchases or sews them herself. He is incapable of getting her to stop interfering. The only way he has of withdrawing from her influence is to stay away from her altogether, as he is unable to stand up to her meddling.

Confronted with her, his feeling of being nobody is the most obvious. He cannot manage to come up with a reasonable argument by which to change her behaviour towards him. She will not listen to him, she does not acknowledge him as an independent, separate individual with a will of his own. Transvestism appears to be a means by which to escape from his mother, at least symbolically – to outdo her by becoming her, or to go one better than her.

This mother only seems to be strong and domineering, but in fact she is narcissistically very vulnerable. She is so lacking in self-esteem that she has to manipulate her child completely in order to be validated by him. Peter's father, a weak man who never interferes to correct his wife, barely ever appears in his story. Just like his father, Peter also has a problem standing his ground with his own wife, and, just like him, he has left the raising of the children to her.

Gradually Peter discovers that he has a fear of not being acknowledged by everyone he meets, although he had decided long before that he had become independent from his mother and her influence. He lives with the constant and anxious tension of whether he will manage to hold his ground, no matter with whom. He always feels frightened and helpless everywhere he goes, all the while putting on a show of great composure, big and solid-looking man as he is.

Peter can only experience others as a threat to his sense of self-worth, and he needs to draw them in by talking a great deal and listening very little, just as his mother does with him. He never feels any fear, although it is quite clearly noticeable to an outsider. It is only during his cross-dressing episodes that he feels he is making himself vulnerable. At the same time, he feels strong and audacious as he parades down the street in his women's clothing and high heels.

Just as he cannot let his mother down, so he is equally unable in the transference to express any negative feelings towards me. He has to keep suggesting that the symbiotic atmosphere he creates is no illusion, while, on the other hand, he starts from a mutual, implicit manipulation, as if this were self-evident.

Mothers and babies

Anyone who treats mothers with young children gains first-hand experience with the development of the symbiotic illusion. It concerns insecure mothers who cannot tolerate their own aggression towards the child. They have to experience everything about the baby and the young child as idyllic, which quite often has little to do with reality, of course. The child's crying and unease mean fear and discomfort for the vulnerable mother. However, she cannot allow herself to feel anger or irritation with her child, which gives her the frightening sense that she is not a good mother. Any activity that is not performed for the sake of the child results in a feeling of guilt. This mother is incapable of leaving the child alone for even a moment. She wants to fuse with the baby, who thus can readily develop a sleep disorder.

When the child does not want to go to sleep, it usually means that it cannot bear being separated form the mother. Such is the case when the mother transmits the feeling to the baby that she cannot for a minute do without him. His not sleeping proves to her that the child needs her, that she must spend the whole night with him, that she should neglect her husband, that she should take the child to their bed to sleep between them, and so forth.

The feeling of not being a good mother generally goes back at least one generation. It is important to introduce the previous generation's mother–daughter relationship into everything under consideration. Quite possibly there already was some hostility to the mother's own mother that had to be covered up with a profession of love. The symbiosis existed already and continues to exist, so that the clinging effect is transferred to the next generation.

Wendy

The idea of the symbiotic phase in the development of the baby originates with the American psychoanalyst and child researcher Margaret Mahler.[3]

She studied mothers and young children but, unfortunately, paid very little attention to fathers – a point to which I will come back later. Subsequently, Mahler cast her light on the mother–daughter relationship.[4] She discovered that a so-called undisturbed symbiotic development does not represent an ideal but leads, instead, to unhealthy, morbid growth. Originally, Mahler derived the term symbiosis and symbiotic phase from research with psychotic children, from where she extrapolated to the normal world of children. In other words, normal development was construed from an unhealthy development. Towards the end of her life Mahler herself realized that this does not tally. Instead of the bliss she at first assumed was there, she discovered that there can be a great deal of hostility at play between mother and child, particularly when the mother uses the child to make herself feel better. In the meantime, the symbiotic phase had become so fashionable that it explained just about every disorder.

However, looking back, as early as 1975, Mahler already gave an outstanding example of a parasitic relationship between a mother and her baby Wendy.[5] The mother in question is passionately in love with her baby and is totally consumed by her. She is extraordinarily vulnerable and is constantly preoccupied with proving to the researchers that she is a perfect mother. Every time the child tries to broaden her social horizon and establish contact with someone other than her mother, the latter immediately goes into action and is possessive where Wendy is concerned. Her child has to validate her by signalling day and night that she needs her. Here Mahler supposes an innate sensitivity on the part of the child, for when she was only 4 months old she was already zooming in on her mother's wishes. The mother was incapable of playfully permitting the baby's individuation. This led to tensions, and the child felt it all too strongly. In my opinion, it seems more likely that the baby learned very early on how to attune herself with all her antennas to the mother's unconscious needs. She sensed the mother's rejection when she would turn away, just as babies are sensitive to all moods.

Later research has proven this 'attunement' of babies. It begins at birth[6] and has little to do with innate aptitude. That is present as well, of course, but what happens in the interaction is equally decisive, actually shaping the final result. This is especially true when it concerns a form of highly distorted emotional interaction.

Wendy cannot play by herself. She tries constantly and desperately to remain the centre of attention and is never happy. What we see here is the beginning of a vulnerable narcissistic personality in a nutshell. The situation is reminiscent of Aïda's, where we saw how even in adulthood mother and daughter maintain a game of mutual dependency. A pattern that provides satisfaction to both is soon formed. The child stimulates the mother to continue her disturbed behaviour. The mother emits signals that she interprets every deviation from her expectations as a rejection, thereby encouraging the child's feelings of guilt.

Wendy showed a vastly diminished need to explore her surroundings because the mother gave nonverbal signs of disapproval as soon as she made such moves. Thus very early on an intense separation anxiety developed. In Wendy an overpowering yearning for closeness ousted all other needs, such as the ability to show an interest in the world around her. Wholly dependent as children are, she learned to show an interest only in those people of whom her mother subtly indicated she approved. She was always busy trying to please her mother, and as a toddler and later as a pre-schooler she did so by going back to the non-verbal intimacy of the mother–baby relationship. When the mother was not there, Wendy was disgruntled and would be pouting angrily – a sign of the paralysing ambivalence in the relationship between the two. Disgruntlement and anger could not be expressed in the mother's presence. Wendy was far too afraid of displeasing her unstable mother and eliciting disapproval. A child is too much in need of the mother's love not to do what the latter wants. Anger only appeared when Wendy was with people other than her mother. This mechanism is known as 'splitting'. The same mechanism applies when children enjoy stories about the hateful stepmother, reserving their love for their own mother. The good and the bad mother – the same person originally – are divided between two or more individuals, so that the positive relationship with the mother is not threatened. When the mother was present, Wendy behaved passively and in baby-like manner. It seemed as if she were clinging to the illusion that she was one with her mother, which is normal only at the beginning of life perhaps and even then only partially or momentarily. At the same time she always feared that her mother would reject her if she did not please her enough. Both mother and child needed constant mutual validation and reassurance.

Wendy was a vulnerable child with low self-esteem and visibly uncertain about her position. The child feels the mother's threatened rejection and reacts to it by adapting. There was a tangible tension between mother and child. When they were together, Wendy gave the impression of being extremely tense. The ambivalence of the frightened and tense mother elicited similar feelings in the child. Wendy tried to escape from her mother's hostility and avert her mother's fear by abandoning her own desire for independence. Mother and daughter thus develop a mirror relationship, for each is dependent on the other for support of her sense of self-worth.

In this way the child develops an 'as-if' personality such as Peter had: someone who tries to fulfil the desires of the other instead of making his own way. As adults such individuals often have no clue as to who they are or what they really want. Their adjustment resembles that of the protagonist in Woody Allen's film *Zelig*: he turns into a Native American among the Native Americans and a Chinese among the Chinese, he is able to take on any colour and attitude he desires. These people are not interested in others as individuals but see them rather as robots that satisfy a need for approval, just as with a vending machine, where you put something in and get something you want in return. These people cannot escape from their narcissistic bastion, their need for attention and validation determines their behaviour.

Not only are unconscious emotions and attitudes of parents reflected in the child's inner tapestry, but their mutual relationship is too. If the mother hates men because she has been deserted by her child's father, she may implant this attitude in the child or project it onto him. Depressive mothers have an overwhelming influence on the mood of their baby, who in turn becomes depressed as well – or hyperactive in order to lure her away from her disconsolate moods. Wendy's case illustrates what happens when symbiosis is created with an actual mutual dependency. This interaction creates not only an illusion but sometimes even a delusion – or in any event a false idyll of consensus – of 'we are alike', of a twosome that will not tolerate a third person. This setting leaves no room for overt resistance or anger, which is ventilated elsewhere outside the dyad and remains unconscious.

Twins

Twins have a psychology that is entirely their own; this has as yet not been sufficiently studied. Being twins is a spontaneously generated, natural symbiosis of two individuals. Sometimes the twin brother or sister compensates for a missing close bond with the mother. Sometimes twins have more to do with each other than with any other person, the mother included. Hate between twins is quite notable as well. Often they cannot stand each other, no matter how much they love one another. They cannot be together, and they cannot do without each other. The separation is often quite dramatic. When they are adults and have to start living their own lives, depression frequently follows. Conversely, sometimes they could happily kill each other.

Usually one of the two represents them both to the outside world, thereby developing more socially and having a bigger mouth. Sometimes that equilibrium is entirely reversed – for instance when the two leave home and have to fend for themselves. Twins often have a hard time when they try to establish their own separate identities. The more introverted one has a greater chance of ending up in psychotherapy. She may belittle herself, for example, and idealize the other, who to the outside world seems to be much more successful yet sometimes turns out to be desperately unhappy.

Frances was extremely jealous of her successful but infertile sister. She decided to be a surrogate mother for her with the semen of her sister's husband. When the child was born, what she had suspected turned out to be true: the child was hers and her husband's, for at around the same time that the insemination had taken place she had also had sexual relations with her husband. Naturally, this had to be kept secret, especially from her sister, to whom she had given the baby in the interim. To make matters worse, she not only felt extremely guilty but, secretly, she also felt triumphant over her twin sister, whom she had managed to really trick for once.

In my office Frances not only came to unload her feelings of worthlessness vis-à-vis her sister, but also her rancour. She betrayed an extremely masochistic, self-deprecating attitude that expressed itself in her whole posture: she sat huddled down like someone who deserves to be punished. She had also entered into a sadomasochistic relationship in which she allowed herself to be humiliated by her lover, a married man. This perverted sexuality serves to dissolve inner tension and give expression to conflicts that have nothing to do with sex. Frances offered herself, not as a person but, rather, as an object with and to which anything can be done. That is how she eradicated her guilt feelings, which must have been present throughout her life, and enjoyed it, to boot. Frances' mother hardly ever appeared in the story. Twins are frequently so completely focused on one another that the mother matters less.

Another woman, Alicia, with a serious borderline disorder, was equally incapable of detaching herself from the relationship with her twin. She was extremely jealous of her more successful sister. At the same time she felt terribly guilty towards her. The cause of this was something that had occurred in their early childhood, had made a deep impression on her, and had serious consequences as well. She had played with matches and had accidentally set fire to her sister's nylon dress. The latter still bore the disfiguring traces of the burns and was visibly wounded. Alicia was emotionally wounded; she was totally paralysed and incapable of making something of her life. She needed to disparage herself constantly and compulsively. This sad woman unconsciously lived with the fear that she was guilty of having attempted to murder her sister, for which she had to pay for the rest of her life.

Well known, too, is the problematic nature of the surviving half of twins, one of whom died either in the womb or just after birth. Frequently the result is a lifelong feeling of guilt. Furthermore, this is often accompanied by a sense – which the parents sowed perhaps – that it is the wrong one who survived. Only good is to be spoken of the dead: that is how dead children are often idealized at the expense of the living.

The symbiotic illusion can be just as invalidating with twins as with mothers and daughters. Jealousy, hate, anger must all be denied or forged into masochism. The feeling of self-worth has no chance of developing if no personality development separate from the other takes place. Just as Siamese twins are physically intertwined, normal twins are psychically interwoven. On rare occasions it really goes wrong, but usually they disentangle spontaneously.

Pia, also a twin, has not developed any symbiosis with her sister. She is actually extremely distant from her – something that is remarkable because it is so rare. This woman has a paranoid mother who always pushed her away, rejected her professions of love, and kept her at a distance. Pia is lesbian and may hope to gather the mother love she so sorely missed that way, after all. She fell deeply in love with her female therapist and got stuck in a feeling of disappointment with life.

I was probably the first person who really listened to her, which in this seriously deprived woman incited slumbering yearnings for motherly love. She saw me, almost in a delusional way, as depressive and needy. I needed her, although I was unwilling to admit it. She had to take care of me, she thought. I could not talk her out of this – a characteristic of delusion. She often felt rejected by me, a repetition in the transference of her experience with her mother's rejecting, even spurning behaviour. Unfortunately, it turned out that little was to be done about it. In Pia, fierce idealization and barely concealed rage alternated.

Symbiotic illusion from generation to generation

The nineteenth-century Dutch writer Louis Couperus in his book *Van oude mensen, de dingen die voorbijgaan* [Of Old People, Things that Pass] clearly proves his insight into the transmission of traumatic events to subsequent generations. Grandma's lover had murdered her husband, and the family has been accursed ever since this secret unspoken episode. Her children and grandchildren all manifest strange symptoms that are linked to the hushed-up killing, and Grandma's never-resolved sense of culpability.

The influences that are transmitted from one generation to the next are extremely conspicuous between mothers and daughters, as has been mentioned before. After all, mothers form an essential connection between generations. Motherhood is at least a three-generational experience that awakens ancient fears and conflicts. The female lineage is the mightiest transmitter of emotional attitudes because of the strong mutual involvement of mothers and daughters plus their gender equivalence. Both fine characteristics and flaws are passed on without the wholesome intervention of the gender difference that helps to acknowledge and allow for differences.

The original homosexual (in the sense of same gender) connection between mothers and daughters does not fail to have an effect on female development.[7] The necessity for a girl to identify with her mother, added to the sameness of sexual and female identity, creates an equivalent orientation and the illusion, which often goes hand in hand, of being the same. To paraphrase Charlotte Gray: 'Daughters and mothers never truly part / Bound in the beating of each other's heart.' There is nothing new here. Nevertheless, one forgets all too often that women can best be considered in the context of preceding and subsequent generations, particularly when there are problems, such as postnatal depression.

An expectant mother sometimes has the fantasy that all her yearnings, aspirations, and unfulfilled ideals will be met by her daughter. When the distance to the actual baby is not too great, the fantasy baby will not get in the way of the reaction to the real baby. But if the mother is very insecure and narcissistically vulnerable, feels threatened in her sense of self-worth, or is depressed, she will not be able to tell her fantasy baby and actual baby apart very well. At that point she sees in the cradle what she hopes to see – or else the one she did not want to see again – instead of the child that is lying there as its own individual being and in its own manifestation.

She sees her despised mother in the baby and reacts by projecting her past onto it: 'She wanted nothing to do with me from the moment she was born', 'She never wanted to be touched', 'She has always been very distant', and so forth. She ignores the child's needs when they are not in keeping with her preconceptions and fears. She sees her baby as her enemy or, conversely, as a part of her body and mind. In the latter case, she will begin to consider her baby as an irreplaceable extension of herself. The child is fed when the mother is hungry or gets attention when she is in need of validation.

All of this occurs more frequently when the mother is insufficiently detached from her own mother. The person a woman carries inside her head is not so much the mother of today but more accurately the image she has shaped around the mother during childhood: the internal mother. That image is only very partially realistic, coloured as it is by the child's fantasy world. Every child within the same family thus has different parents because it has experienced those parents in its own personal way.

The narcissistically insecure new mother sees her child as her enemy unless it satisfies her needs. That is why she is unable to permit anything resembling separation or individuation. The bond with her own mother was never loosened enough to make another relationship wholly possible. She may well be married, have a husband or partner or a special female friend, but an invisible umbilical cord still links her to her mother. She has remained dyadic rather than grown to be triadic – that is to say, the third person who might have intervened, the father, has in her experience been missing too much.

Just as her father played a small part in her life, so the partner's place is unclear to her as well. He has a limited role. Her attitude is not especially heterosexual. After the birth of their child, such a woman often no longer has any interest whatsoever in a sexual relationship. She tends to be totally absorbed in her baby and has lost interest in the outside world. Her partner might even be blamed for disrupting the bond with the mother, the child, or a woman friend.

As we saw earlier, the mother and daughter's being shackled to one another is a source of frustration and aggression that does not disappear when the daughter herself becomes a mother. One or the other gets the short end of the stick: if I detach myself, things will end badly for me, or my mother will fall apart. In its many variations 'Either my mother or I, one of us will die', is a frequently expressed fantasy. The autonomy of one is life-threatening for the other. Sometimes the father becomes the bad guy about whom the mother gossips to her daughter, which is how they manage to maintain the peace between them.

Mother and daughter have a negotiated agreement in which they apply the 'one good turn deserves another' approach. It is clearly a kind of barter.[8]

When the signs indicating that 'I need you' are not forthcoming, symbiotic love can easily turn into blind hatred. The mother drops the daughter. Sometimes it is the daughter who moves away. Her fear of being swallowed up leads to a kind of symbiosis phobia: stay as far away from your mother as you can, especially when you've just given birth. She might steal or destroy the child out of pure jealousy, just as the wicked fairy does in some fairy tales. The loss of their own identity when mother comes anywhere near her creates panic in these daughters.

In men the symbiosis with their mother leads to a threat to their sexual identity. After all, the man is then supposed to resemble her, to feel and think the same things as her. This means that he has to be a woman with women, so that he might like being with them but will avoid them as sexual partners. Or else he may have a female partner and seek refuge in strange sexual scenarios. That is where he plays out the threat of being swallowed up by the mother or of turning into a woman. In sadomasochistic sexual scenarios the fear of castration is merely acted out in fantasy play. Fright and excitement then come together in the flush of victory known as orgasm.

Such perverse – in the sense of reality turned upside down – sexual scenarios have a dreamlike quality, and for their meaning they have to be interpreted as the dream texts that they are. The latent significance lies hidden behind the manifest content. Although certainly not unknown, this kind of scenario is much less common in women. Women have a different kind of fear of castration from men but are no less anxious about injury to the inside of their body, or even complete destruction caused by their imaginary mother, who then resembles the wicked witch of the fairy tales.

When a daughter becomes pregnant, she sometimes senses two competing dyads arising. She must be loyal to her mother but also has her child to care for. She is called on from two sides. The grandmother and the baby are fighting for the young mother's attention. She fears her mother's jealousy of the child who is now getting her full attention. Then she begins to suffer great strain, and will become depressed and furious, usually with her husband. No matter how hard he tries, he can never do anything right any more.

The woman with a postnatal depression solves her painful dilemma by really starting to hate her mother, her child, or herself. If she hates her baby but cannot tolerate this hatred because of her feelings of guilt, so she will try her utmost to take extra good care of the child. That way she forms a barrier against her own murderous tendencies. She becomes overprotective, has no time for herself, and cannot leave the baby alone. The baby's crying means an accusation of her as a bad mother. Besides, she feels an intense longing to be a baby herself and be attended to by a loving mother.

Lea has severe postnatal depression. She feels her mother is overbearing, intrusive, and meddling. At the same time, she suggests that there is something very special between her mother and herself. The ambivalence is therefore very obvious. It is as if she is living in two separate worlds, as if her mind is split into two separate halves. In the one half her mother is very intimate and close, in the other she senses the lack of a mother who is supportive. When I ask her what the good contact with her mother consists of, she becomes sad and has no answer. The illusion is painfully disrupted by reflecting upon it.

Actually, her mother mostly complains while Lea listens, hiding her annoyance. She is still hoping for those delightful moments that could be, but that never appear. Her wish to be one with her mother is only kept in check by the fear that her mother will take over her life and that she will be driven off course. For instance, when her mother says how much she likes her son-in-law, Lea suddenly cannot stand her husband any more. Her mother's wish should not become hers in any way whatsoever, or else she will have no personal life left. 'My mother swallows me up, it seems as if I completely vanish.' This combination of a lifelong yearning for and an always-returning disappointment in the mother is not unusual in women.

It is difficult to abandon lifelong desires and yearnings and to realize that they will never come to be. Lea's mother can never be any support to her because she cannot bear it when Lea is having a hard time. It makes her feel sick herself. It is a topsy-turvy relationship in which her mother is constantly appealing to her. In her own eyes, she must unconditionally support her mother. Negative feelings are directed outside the dyad towards the excluded third person, the father. According to Lea, a true dialogue in which she will be listened to is impossible. Her preoccupations do not really matter to her mother, who is too concerned with her own sense of being neglected. This has its reason: she herself was an abandoned child. (Chapter 7 deals more extensively with postnatal depression.)

Sandra is another example of the multigenerational problem. She complains that her mother will not listen and only talks about herself. She hates her mother intensely and does not know how to handle this. As an adolescent she had been institutionalized because of manifestations of a severe obsessive-compulsive disorder, accompanied by delusions and fears. Despite a successful career, she still suffers from a delusional asbestos phobia. She is constantly afraid she will step on asbestos and then contaminate everyone around her. She worries about this for hours on end. She knows it is not true, and yet she believes it. I ask her to bring her mother, and on that occasion I see that, indeed, the mother does not listen, does not want to hear about Sandra's complaints, puts a positive label on everything, acts nice in an inadequate manner, while her daughter is clearly annoyed and then depressed. Sandra just sits there, her head down, looking more and more like a broken flower.

The mother's prehistory explains a few things. She was an unwanted child and the loveless relationship between her and her own mother has now led to the unacknowledged hate between her and her daughter. While the mother tries to sweettalk and cover up her hate, the daughter barely manages to do so. The obsessive asbestos story can be interpreted as 'ash-best'. Mother – who has a piece of asbestos in her collection of fossils – could only turn into ashes herself. Sandra cannot possibly admit to such a wish, although she admits that she does not love her mother and, in fact, loathes her. She is weighed down by feelings of guilt about all sorts of trivial inanities but, in all likelihood, due to her murderous fantasies that are not allowed to become conscious.

Music is a suitable medium in which to become lost. Clara Schumann, the wife of the composer Robert Schumann, was a renowned nineteenth-century pianist. Because of her parents' divorce she lost her mother when she was quite young. She stayed behind with a harsh father who loved her on condition that she achieved what he wanted. Yet, she was capable of experiencing moments of bliss. Presumably, she managed to hold on to a good feeling from the time she had shared with her mother. When the latter, a gifted pianist and singer, accompanied herself on the piano, little Clara used to sit under the piano and listen.[9]

In conclusion

Symbiosis literally means the mutual dependency of two organisms. This biological concept is used here in its psychological meaning and refers to the inhibiting mutual dependency of two individuals – specifically, the parasitic relationship between parent, mostly the mother, and her child. Hostility between the two is held at bay, while all anger and aggression can conveniently be projected on a third person outside the dyad, usually the father.

Symbiosis is an emotional situation that appears momentarily and provides a feeling of bliss. We rediscover this feeling of momentary bliss, which originates in the period of babyhood, when we look at art, a beautiful landscape, or in an intimate contact such as being in love.

A complete lack of emotional closeness is just as traumatic as its opposite: a quasi-intimacy without boundaries where any separation is disavowed. Living without illusions is as distressing as drowning in them.

The ability to love – a blissful emotion – goes back to our first experiences with the mother. A daughter need not renounce her mother in order to become independent. On the contrary, the daughter will end up in trouble in the case of an extreme solution in one direction or the other – whether she flees from or rejects her mother in an attempt to gain independence, or whether she keeps clinging to her, thinking she must take care of her, protect her. Some women grow up without a mother and continue to feel a painful loss forever. Some mothers die or abandon their offspring, or have so many children that they cannot pay attention to each one of them individually. A total lack of any symbiotic experience causes as much of a void as an excessive fusing with a love object. Fortunately, we see a happy medium in the majority of cases. The mother serves as an example for her daughter, gives her a feeling of support, and helps her to become a mother herself.

The role played by the mother's unconscious has long been ignored. Sigmund Freud showed very little interest in mothers. The lack of interest among the pioneers of psychoanalysis – with the exception of Helene Deutsch[10] – in the role of the mother has had far-reaching consequences. The mother–daughter relationship and, for example, the postnatal depression connected with it thus remained unsolved. The father, who held a central place for the creator of psychoanalysis and his early followers, here remained mostly out of sight in the work of subsequent researchers. By contrast, Melanie Klein, Anna Freud, and Margaret Mahler, among others, gave a more central place to the mother and the earliest stages of development.

Chapter 3

History of maternal love

There is nothing either good or bad,
But thinking makes it so.
William Shakespeare

Some historical awareness is required for us to understand our own world-view and put it into perspective. First let us look at the position that mothers and children have held throughout the centuries; it will then be shown that the norm has shifted from a relative neglect of children in large paternalistic families to an often exclusive bond with the mother figure.

If maternal love had always been self-evident, then why would it have been demanded of mothers? It is important to realize that encouragement towards greater maternal love has only been prevalent for a few hundred years.[1]

Imposing requirements on mothers began with the Enlightenment. Apparently, these new moral principles were needed because all too frequently it was neglect and a lack of interest in the child that was the norm. Too many children died too young. This was detrimental to the economy: with the advent of the industrial revolution, ever more manual labour was needed.

Relationships between parents and children are strongly determined by time and place – that is to say, not only by the culture of a region, a social class, an ethnic group, but also by the historical moment. If we want to examine motherhood in the Western world more closely, we also have to look at the past and at the genesis of the concept of maternal love, which is not self-evident in the least.

In north-western Europe and America more psychosocial changes have occurred in the last two centuries than ever before in history. The *ancien régime* – the period preceding the French Revolution – was gone forever. Indeed, although the new era first and foremost benefited the bourgeoisie while the rest of the population did not come to enjoy more favourable circumstances until much later, yet a noticeable change in mentality was taking place. Obviously, the new attitude towards children had major consequences, not only for their everyday living conditions but also for their inner lives.

Since the eighteenth century, maternal love has been getting more attention than ever before. Because of the industrial revolution and urbanization, in particular, when home and work became separated, the mother acquired the central place for the child, and her task lay within the family. The family became a kind of safe haven,[2] a world apart.[3] As we shall see, in the nineteenth century the special interest in the raising of children actually develops into all sorts of frightening preoccupations.[4]

After 1900 the interest in childhood expands further and takes a different direction, partly as a result of Sigmund Freud's discoveries. Psychoanalysis stimulates the interest in the feelings and fantasies of the child. Furthermore, after the end of the Second World War, an entirely new tendency arises as a result of greater clarity around the traumas of loss, separation, and abandonment. The exclusivity and intensity of the mother–child relationship gains ever more emphasis in mental health care. Maternal care, the highest good for which to strive, grows into a new ethics.[5]

Ever since the popularization of psychoanalysis, maternal love has become the concern of all responsible parents. Growing and increasing knowledge of early childhood development has been helpful for parents but has also made them – mothers in particular – more anxious and guilt-ridden. The current era belongs in a vaster historic movement that has been going on for a much longer time. How did all this come about?

Psychosocial history and the history of mentality tell us about the ways of thinking and the everyday life of both our close and our distant ancestors. Various new sources of research have been tapped: visual material such as old paintings and prints, church registers, legal judgments, last wills and testaments, diaries, letters, physicians, and midwives' notes. All these sources are a goldmine that historians did not discover until rather late in the day, when they began to grow tired of kings and generals as the only interesting figures of our past. Then the advent of the computer made demographic material truly accessible, whereby historical reflection became democratized.

Thus informed about our past, it is really only now that we are able to compare our way of life with that of bygone eras, just as anthropology was previously able to compare us and our distant and not so distant forebears. By means of what can be found in the historic literature,[6] I shall attempt to ascertain how parents used to behave and feel towards their children in earlier times. Comparisons between bygone days and today put the obvious into perspective because it becomes clearer to us that each era has its own approach.

The question is how the modern standard of the exclusivity of maternal love relates to psychic health. Exclusivity makes stringent requirements on the quality of the relationship. The mother's emotional health becomes a decisive factor when the care and rearing of the child is primarily left up to her. It is precisely because the role – indeed, the indispensability – of the father is all too frequently overlooked that the way towards pathology may be paved.

Maternal love before the eighteenth century

The history of maternal love can be roughly divided into two periods. The second of these made a cautious start in the second half of the seventeenth century. It was at that time that maternal love first became a philosophical ideal, a goal to aspire to, and a topic of manuals on morality and child-rearing. In the eighteenth century these concepts were increasingly put into practice. Generally speaking, before that time maternal love had no more been a topic of discussion than sexuality ever was. Especially for the poor, children were a burden rather than a treasure. In this context the Dutch statesman and popular poet 'Father Cats' (Jacob Cats, 1577–1660) comes to mind, whom my mother liked to quote when she was annoyed with us: 'Children are hindrances', she would say.

However, it is true that historians are divided in their views on maternal love. There are proponents and opponents of the pioneer Philippe Ariès, who was the first to describe childcare under the *ancien régime*. According to him, the child had been treated better in the Middle Ages than later on, when strict and often harsh Protestantism had entered the stage. Nevertheless, in Ariès' opinion, children in bygone days generally received very little special atten-tion. Society was a colourful mixture of ranks and classes in which everyone knew his God-given place. Although children and adults did spend time in each other's company, there was no particular interest in the experiences of the child.

The historian Emmanuel Le Roy Ladurie disagrees.[7] He describes the mountain village Montaillou in the Pyrenees on the basis of archives from the Inquisition. The Cathars of that region were cruelly persecuted as heretics and punished accordingly. According to Ladurie, they were kind and caring in dealing with their children, however. Two brief comments should be made in this context. It may be that in southern Europe different customs – that is to say, gentler and more child-friendly ones – were the rule rather than those in areas farther north. On the other hand, one could surmise that the sadism of the Inquisitors and the asceticism of the Cathar heretics would inspire great toughness in them. It is well known that the Cathars were quite ascetic – in the sexual sphere, for example – and that women were merely second-rate citizens. One would assume that all of this must have had something to do with their upbringing.

Another French study also disagrees with Ariès. The authors, Pierre Richier and Danièle Alexandre-Bidon, demonstrate with visual material that attention was most definitely being paid to the interest of the child. People exerted themselves to promote development by means of a great deal of attention, and with children's toys, above all.[8] The group of historians known as the Cambridge Group[9] saw a clear difference between north-western Europe, where children were always in a better position, and the rest of the world. They posit that the nuclear family and the intimacy it can provide have always existed in certain regions, such as in England. They believe that in the time of Julius Caesar the Gauls may already have been familiar with a nuclear family and were far more child-friendly than the ruthless Romans.

The above-mentioned historians disagree with Ariès' model of evolution. They do not see a gradual change from bad to better but assume that there have always been vast regional differences. The 'crude barbarians' were actually less hard and cruel to their children and more interested in family life than were the Romans. In the classical world, for instance, there was no equivalent for the word *baby*, and the word *discipline* was literally synonymous with punishment. Children, women, and slaves all held a similarly marginal position in ancient society. That situation did not change until the arrival of Christianity. No matter how the above-mentioned discussion about childhood in earlier times may be settled, specific knowledge of the child has in large measure been lacking until the advent of psychoanalysis.

The hopeful model of development that includes progress looks less probable to me. It seems to be primarily based on factors such as time, place, economy, and national character. This is illustrated by the fact that in many Third World areas children are currently still badly treated. Some cultures, like the Protestant countries of the north, have a tendency to improve by hard work, by making use of the human potential, by creating privacy, or by expanding mutually dependent human relationships into greater intimacy. Other cultures may never head in that direction.

The historian Lloyd deMause, although he certainly has not gone unchallenged, is sombre about the past: 'The history of childhood is a nightmare from which we're only recently beginning to awaken.'[10]

As circumstances rendered people's destiny harder and sadder, they treated their children more ruthlessly. The desperately poor have always aborted, killed, or abandoned, their children, or sold them to be handed over to a life of prostitution. In the Third World that is still happening today. Early parental death has also often resulted in children being left to their fate.

Infanticide was relatively common in antiquity, specifically in Greece. Remember Agamemnon, who first murdered Clytemnestra's baby before he would marry her and then sacrificed his daughter Iphigenia to the gods to negotiate fortunate winds for his fleet. The Old Testament, too, tells of a myriad infanticides, even though Isaiah strictly forbade it. Think of Abraham, who placed his son Isaac on the sacrificial stone to placate his God. The Celts and the Germanic tribes also practiced infanticide. Child sacrifice was generally rationalized as the will of the gods. Often it was practised as a form of birth control after birth.

Lack of food, incompetence in the face of procreation, and a preference for sons have always led to the overt or masked killing of children. This still happens in India and in China. Judaism maintains the sacrifice of the foreskin as a *pars pro toto* symbol of the whole child. In primal times, sacrificing the firstborn son to the almighty deity was apparently a duty, though it could sometimes be discharged by using animals instead. This was the case with Abraham, who, in the end, sacrifices a ram instead of his son Isaac. Christianity actually uses the sacrifice of the son as a fundamental myth and as a metaphor for divine mercy. In the Middle Ages, from approximately the fourth century onwards, the Church resisted the blatant killing of children. The custom was more or less officially brought to an end in the fifteenth century. Infanticide, having now become a crime, was subsequently projected onto the Jews, a tall story that can still be heard today in the countryside of Austria, for example; the ambivalence that children evoke survives until today.

Abandoning a child as a foundling was long a conventional means of getting rid of undesired progeny. In the Middle Ages some 20–40 per cent of all children were aborted, killed, or abandoned as foundlings.[11] In the eighteenth century, the abandonment of foundling children and putting them up with a wet nurse again increased vastly in Europe's poor Roman Catholic area, despite the official line of the Church that fought it strongly. In Vienna, in the early nineteenth century, as many as 50 per cent of all children were abandoned as foundlings.[12] Infant corpses were found with great regularity in the gutter or on rubbish heaps in nineteenth-century London. Due to the population growth, the demographics changed, and children formed a much larger part of the population. The result was that penniless gangs of robbing and stealing children made the large cities unsafe, as still happens in South America today.

Abandoning children as foundlings did not come to an end in France until around 1900. Although once charitable institutions were established children could be left in orphanages or foundling homes, this did not in the least increase their chances for survival. The mortality rate in such institutions was higher than 90 per cent. Even in the friendly Netherlands, where, generally speaking, the circumstances were better than in the rest of the world, the situation for children in such homes was appalling. Indeed, separate foundling homes hardly existed there because foundlings were not as numerous as in other places, but the orphanages treated their pupils harshly. They were severely disciplined and often beaten. For instance, as late as 1661, a law had to be written in Leiden prohibiting orphans from working more than 15 hours a day. In 1671, 8,000 child labourers were still imported to work in the textile industry there, where they functioned pretty much as slaves.

A different way of coping with an overabundance of children was boarding a child out to a paid wet nurse. For centuries, the children of affluent and urban parents, as well as those of poor mothers who had to work to earn their bread, were put out to board with women who, obviously, were even more wretched. If the child survived at all, it would spend anywhere from two to five years with the family of the wet nurse. Such a foster home was usually far from their own abode, in the 'healthy' countryside, where the children's parents would visit them rarely, if ever, during that time. The trip to such a faraway wet nurse was no fun for anyone in those days, but for a newborn it was frequently fatal. Hygiene was not of a high level anywhere, but among the destitute wet nurses it was downright abysmal. Eyewitnesses speak of stench, filth, vermin, and lack of light and air. Just as in the orphanages, the mortality rate among these infants was at least 90 per cent.

When children came home from such a foster family, they obviously did not know their parents at all. They had become strangers who could help or serve their parents. Around 8–10 years old, they might be boarded elsewhere as servants or apprentices to other people totally unknown to them, who often treated them with harshness.

Especially in the upper classes, it was an unpopular concept to have the mother breastfeed the newborn baby herself. Breastfeeding is associated with tenderness, intimacy, and sexuality. Thus, it was seen not only as a burden, but as a dirty and sinful business, too – a wickedness that had better be avoided or left to the inferior classes. However, that was risky also. Superstition around babies and nursing reigned supreme. The child would resemble the one who nursed it, so it was thought. It might ingest bad blood from a malicious wet nurse or adopt the urges of the animal whose milk it had drunk. The composer Wolfgang Amadeus Mozart wrote in 1793: '*Nun hat das Kind wider meinen Willen, und doch mit meinem Willen, eine Saug-Amme bekommen. Meine Frau, sei es imstande oder nicht, sollte niemals ihr Kind stillen, das war immer mein fester Vorsatz! Allein, einer andern Milch soll mein Kind auch nicht hineinschlucken!, sondern bei Wasser, wie meine Schwester und ich, will ich es aufziehen.*' [Now the child has acquired, against my will and yet according to my will, a wet nurse. My wife, whether she were able to or not, would never nurse her child, that was always my firm intention! However, the milk of another should my child also not swallow! but with water, as my sister and I were, will I bring it up.][13]

Additionally, one of the reasons for hiring a wet nurse was that as yet no replacement for breastfeeding existed. The dilemma of feeding an infant effectively other than by nursing would remain unsolved for a long time to come. Not until the end of the nineteenth century did the technique of artificial feeding come into being, and only then did the use of animal milk become popular. Previously, the baby was often given food that was too heavy and indigestible for it.

It was not uncommon for children and adults to sleep in the same bed, and it might happen that one of the parents rolled on top of the baby, thereby suffocating it. Poor farmers' children would be left alone after being swaddled and tied to a small board while their parents worked the land to harvest the crops. That way they could hang the baby on a hook on the wall, not able to move and therefore unable to get into trouble or have an accident. Thus they were safe from rats or dogs, though not from insects or the threat of fire. Freezing or burning to death was not an unusual occurrence.

Infant death was common. Children faced death from a very young age on, accustomed as they were to their little brothers or sisters dying. What we call 'traumatic' today, such as being the 'replacement child', was perfectly normal in earlier times. Parents often gave the same name to consecutive children in the hope that there would be at least *one* John or Peter to be the surviving heir. Children stayed alive only by the will of God, and heaven was not all that bad, anyway. Dying was such a common phenomenon that the dead child was frequently not even mourned.

Minimal bonding between parent and child more or less had to be the result of this ever-threatening loss. The child was idealized in the adoration of the Infant Jesus and as *putti*, angels symbolic of the soul after death, which *adorned* ceilings. That ideal image sadly did not always refer to flesh-and-blood children, nor did it produce any greater empathy for children. Neither did it prevent bad characteristics from being projected onto the child. The contrast lay between the deified and the vilified child.

Violence against children was a normal phenomenon and part of everyday practice. Raising a child properly meant being ruthless in order to suppress the child's innately sinful character. In the fourth century CE, Saint Augustine of Hippo, also known as the Church Father Augustine (354–430), author of the *Confessions*, was one of the first to pay some attention to mothers and children. He believed that the latter ought to be dealt with harshly.[14]

The Reformation always extolled the family as an important institution. Combined with the recent ideas about original sin and personal responsibility, this belief ensured strictness, ruthlessness, and asceticism towards children. Pedagogues advised that the rod should not be spared. Children ought not to be shown any mercy – on the contrary, without beatings they could not be tamed into becoming well-adjusted adults. Punishment and thrashing could not start early enough, for the younger the child, the more obstreperous and malicious it was. Violence against children could also be induced by poverty. Mutilating children, as still occurs in some underdeveloped countries today, served to turn them into beggars later on.

There are many similarities as well as obvious differences between what we know today as underdeveloped countries and our own medieval past. Deficiency and want are the same everywhere, but deliberate severity is a pedagogical method. It is a principle that can obstruct spontaneous affection for the child. It is self-evident that such a form of pedagogy has consequences for the possibility of expressing positive emotions between parents and children. It obviously influenced spontaneous maternal love in a negative way. There is a clear connection between pedagogical styles and national character.

The Japanese national character offers a well-known example. The harshness of the Japanese is sometimes ascribed to the sudden reversal in the way young children are raised. Little children are spoiled and coddled a great deal, but as soon as they are a bit older, this changes abruptly. From the age of 5 onward they are treated with severity, and high demands are made of them. School and having to achieve turn into a veritable torture. For us the rigorous approach towards children, which came with the Reformation, began to be part of the norm around the sixteenth century. The success of the Western world is sometimes attributed to this characteristic, where nothing is left to chance and people are expected to give their utmost, just as Calvinism prescribes. However, opinions vary widely on this matter. The historian Alan MacFarlane[15] challenges the idea that it is the Protestant ethic that furthered Western mentality and prosperity. He indicates a reverse process: the English character was modern even before the Reformation, a bourgeois mentality concerned with duties and hard work had always been prevalent. This is why Puritanism had easier access in these regions and in America than elsewhere.

Fear of catastrophes, disaster, ignorance, and impotence against the natural environment led to magic and superstition. One example of this is the branding of children with blazing pokers to 'protect' them against epilepsy. Babies were submerged in ice-cold water when baptized or else rolled in the snow. Thus the child frequently contracted pneumonia and then died of the consequences. Exorcism was normal, certainly before the Reformation, and to exorcise the devil it was a good sign when the child cried loudly and long during baptism.

Babies are not merely adorable, but they are also a burden. Not infrequently, the pressure on the parents causes an unconscious hatred towards the child. In our day aggression against children has become a taboo, so that it is only a disturbed parent who knowingly harms a child. In bygone days that worked quite differently. Babies might be rocked so roughly that they would become unconscious, just to get them to be quiet and fall asleep. A wad with something sweet or even with opium or alcohol was put into their mouths to keep them calm.

The concept that children are supposed to be hardened continues even today. In the past, pampering was wicked and hardening was often taken quite literally. This was done by means of much whipping, little food, rough and indigestible fare, without tenderness or any form of affectionate physical contract. Hard beds, cold rooms, scarce meals – such was the lot of the child. Their clothes had to be made of coarse fabric, simple and chaste, and preferably not too warm. In winter children were quite frequently unprotected from the fierce cold. From the sixteenth century onward, these kinds of measures were systematically recommended by both physicians and pedagogues like Jean-Jacques Rousseau.

For the most part, girls were given even less to eat than boys; they were valued less and their mere survival was deemed to be sufficient.[16] Girls learned little, so education was not considered to be necessary for them; it was not worth all the investment. They needed to learn household tasks. In the non-Western world this remains unchanged and is still in effect today. Even in the Western world the generation of women who were not permitted to get an education is still not extinct.

For a long time everything that verged on gentleness and tenderness towards children was suspect – almost the reverse of the maternal love educators and psychologists recommend today. In aristocratic circles, the pedagogical precepts of the philosophers, who had been writing about childrearing for centuries, were less compelling. Other, private norms held sway there, and it was important, for instance, to have good manners, to take part in hunting, and to be able to ride. Louis XIII, a royal prince, was raised in an exemplary fashion. He had to learn to play the violin at 3 years of age. When disobedient, though, he was lashed into submission or threatened with whipping, which, according to his personal physician, caused him nightmares.[17]

When children did not obey, they had to be browbeaten. Well into the nineteenth century, this was done by way of ghost- and horror stories, while hell and damnation were used as threats. Even in the twentieth century some educators would still use masks to strike the necessary fear into children. The child was especially not permitted to have a will of its own, which had to be 'broken' each time it raised its undesirable head. According to the moralists, only bad parents treated their child with gentleness. Mothers, in particular, were blamed for this evil. 'Spare the rod and spoil the child', was a popular saying. Schreber, one of Sigmund Freud's famous case studies,[18] was the son of a well-known pedagogue whose brutality left his son with a severe case of paranoia.[19]

Swaddling babies day and night, making them into an easily manageable package, which is still commonly done in Russia and parts of Eastern Europe, has been practised for thousands of years. Apparently, free movement was considered dangerous. The child was weak and fragile by nature and ought not only to be kept to the straight and narrow path, but also needed to be kept literally upright. The result was a moral and physical straitjacket. Swaddling made any spontaneous interaction with the mother impossible, although she apparently felt little need for it herself. The child dared not make a move and was forced into passivity with all the emotional consequences thereof. Crawling was not recommended, because it was too reminiscent of the animal world. The child had to walk right from the word go, which could be arranged with the aid of a small rolling cart on wheels. But this was a luxury.

For a long time, child labour was very common. As mentioned before, children were raised outside the parental home, usually from their tenth year onward and sometimes earlier. Parents would 'exchange' their children to have them work as servants. Often children became apprentices for a boss who would teach them a vocation or a craft. They were to become involved in the working world as quickly as possible.[20] In the Third World, children are made available from about the age of 4 on to do work that is often much too hard for them, such as hauling stones. In antiquity children would be sold as slaves, a custom that in Italy continued well into the Renaissance. The exploitation of children began long before the advent of industrial revolution and capitalism.

Until the eighteenth century, no great attention was paid to the subject of children and sexuality. The smallest ones were handled very freely. However, from the age of 7 on, greater discipline and a certain amount of modesty from and towards the child were seen as important. From then on, the child was no longer the exclusive responsibility of its mother and the other women in the family. After the Renaissance, in particular, the father became an increasingly more central figure. Although in small form, the child was considered to be an adult from its seventh year onward, at which point boys were brought into male society.

For a long time the division within the community and housing arrangements were such that children were aware of the actions and experiences of adults. Sexuality did not become a secret until the invention of the nursery and the concept of privacy, a result of the changing mores. Spontaneous sexual expressions of children or adults were not yet a separate point of focus, and certainly not a specific problem. Sexual contact with children was nothing special in ancient Greece or Rome. Anal contact with little boys and fellatio of the adult male by the little boy were extremely popular. This can be observed into the Renaissance on a large scale. It took Christianity to introduce the need for the child's sexual 'innocence', an idea that met with little response in everyday practice.

Magic around sexuality and around the unresolved mysterious problems of contagious diseases is reflected in the prevailing superstition. The feared venereal diseases could be prevented or even cured, they thought, by having intercourse with an 'innocent' child. Currently, ever younger girls are popular as prostitutes to provide protection against, or even cure, AIDS in Third World countries.

We find a touching example of childhood liberties, but also of adult handling of the child as a kind of wind-up doll, in the journals of Jean Héroard, the court physician of the royal prince Louis XIII. As a toddler, around the year 1600, little Louis was allowed to freely show his 'guillery' and let all the courtiers touch and kiss it. The boundaries of modesty were raised to the present level only very gradually and relatively late.[21] The little prince would frolic naked in bed with his parents, playing with the queen's breasts, while the court physician watched and noted everything down for posterity.

The concept of maternal love is a result of the modernization process. The fact that a child needs love, care, and empathy is a recent notion. Before the eighteenth century one did not try to put oneself in the shoes of the child but expected precocious behaviour from it, adapted to adults. The personality of a child was never connected to pedagogical methods – all its characteristics were attributed to heredity or to its intrinsic nature. Yet, the famous Dutch historian Johan Huizinga already pointed out to what extent the cruel and harsh treatment of children turned them into cruel and suspicious adults.[22]

There was hardly any question of a separate child's world as we know it today, even though the concept was not completely missing. Some form of the child's world and of specific child's play can already be noted in the Middle Ages. Adults were more childlike and believed in fairy tales, just as today's children do. Adults projected with even greater ease than they do today. Undesirable impulses were rather quickly ascribed to children, witches, outsiders, or strangers. Fears, too, were lavishly projected onto children. Anxiety about the satanic, attributed chiefly to small children, was widespread, sometimes with tragic results.

People believed in magic, similar to those who in some places still believe in faith healers now. This also meant that impulses of love and hate, feelings of sorrow and fear, were given freer rein. The child was not much more than a serf, a slave, a spineless projection screen. The parent often expected it to provide help, support, care, and love. If it could not satisfy these expectations, its life might even be at stake, something that we now call child abuse or exploitation. The child could easily be blamed for the fears and ailments from which the parents suffered, such as the often acute food shortages. Fairy tales such as Little Tom Thumb and Hansel and Gretel are reminders thereof. They were literally sent off into the forest because there was no food for them at home any more. They simply had to fend for themselves or else die of starvation, like the street urchins of today.

Superstition was rampant in a world that could often be unstable or menacing. Unconditional parental love, loving children and investing in them had not yet been raised to a standard. It was not really possible either because of the child mortality rate, which was so high that people frequently did not even attend the funeral. Parents loved their children in a different way from the way they do in today's small families.

As we have seen, regional differences ought not to be underestimated. The traditional agrarian cultures were and are particularly dependent on children and child labour, which encourages the 'extended family' and large numbers of children. The situation in north-western Europe was different. In those areas the families were smaller, husband and wife were more equal to one another, the freedom of choice of a partner was greater, and the child was more independent than elsewhere.[23]

Especially England, but the Netherlands, too, was already fairly prosperous and far advanced in the process of modernization compared to southern, middle, and eastern Europe. In Holland, the nuclear family was identified as early as the fourteenth century, in England already in the thirteenth century, but it may well have existed long before then. Prosperity and individualism were linked to the more constitutional forms of government in these countries as opposed to the absolute monarchies in power elsewhere. Already there was civil law, a political and economic system, and some curtailment of violence. This differed vastly from the arbitrariness, the Inquisition, and the justice by torture that existed elsewhere in Europe.

Moreover, individualism and freedom of choice were the result of inheritance according to primogeniture, according to the birthright by which the oldest son inherits the land. As an individual, he was free to own and sell that land. Thus the son became independent of his father and freed from the ancient *'patria potestas'*, the power of the father. Sons were also quick to leave home and find their own way in the world, independent of their fathers. They were able to invest their own money and do business as they saw fit.[24] This created strong, resilient people and promoted individualism. In the end, the previously described transformations of the eighteenth century, the industrial and social evolution, as well as the French Revolution, led to the middle-class nuclear family as we still know it today. During the period discussed so far, in which the old regime held sway and tradition had the upper hand, the child grew up more in the community than alone with its parents. Maternal love was not yet an isolated concept, and the exclusivity of the mother–child relationship barely existed.

Although the civilizing process cannot be seen as a linear evolution, nor is it the same as progress, many changes for the better can be observed where children are concerned, at least in the Western world. Generally speaking, the Westerner has been partly domesticated. He has acquired a more uncompromising conscience. When he wants to get something done, he does not immediately resort to brute force: he observes the laws of the land and the demands of his inner regulator, his conscience.[25] That which used to take place in the outside world and was reflected in fairy tales (which were not at all intended for small children only, certainly not in their unexpurgated pre-eighteenth-century form), was replaced by the inner world of people. Not only is violence taboo, it is also prohibited and controlled by the state. Our dreams and fantasies are generally the only – usually unconscious – evidence of our potential for violence. However, the temporary return of the repressed, whether in collective or individual form, does not produce any less horrendous consequences these days. 'Man-made disaster' has not disappeared. There is still no scarcity of overt violence, and the mass consumption of extremely sadistic and violent films and videos gives us cause to suspect the worst where concealed desires are concerned.

Not only was the relationship between parents and children very different from what we have today, but the same was true for conjugal partners as well. Most people married someone chosen or approved by their father. Freedom of choice was much more common in Protestant countries such as England and the northern Netherlands than elsewhere. By and large, however, a marriage was not a personal decision but, rather, one based on tradition and class. The family's material interests superseded any emotional considerations. Although romantic love, whose praises were sung by the troubadours and described by the Swiss writer Denis de Rougemont,[26] has always existed as a concept, love or falling in love were more the exception than the rule. This is still true in the more traditional societies, where parents arrange their children's marriages.

During the *ancien régime* a household was much more an economic unit than an emotional one. In traditional society there is very little latitude for the individual. Expressing individual desires and yearnings was to a great extent unknown. Everyone knew his place in the community, fulfilled his function, and played the role that Providence had assigned to him. Just as the man owed obedience to the king and to God, so the woman – hierarchically on the same level as the children – owed obedience to her husband. The husband sat in judgement upon his wife and children, the same way as the courts of justice do for us. He was at liberty to punish them, discipline them, or even lock them up.

Not only did the wife have no voice, she was also more a mother to her children and performed manual labour in service to her husband than she was his lover. Sexuality served the purpose of procreation, which could be both a blessing and a curse. Awareness of personal sexuality and of the right to express emotional wishes seem to have developed hand in hand with maternal love.

Maternal love from the eighteenth century onwards

As far as one can gather, in the eighteenth century a ground-breaking revolution took place in the life of the emotions. It concerns the same historical movement as the one from which the Reformation grew forth: the modernization process of the middle class. At this time and in this class, the mother definitively became the dominant figure in the child's life. The eighteenth century saw the publication of *Emile* and *La nouvelle Héloïse*, two treatises on education by Jean-Jacques Rousseau, philosopher of the Enlightenment. Moralists were writing admonishing treatises on the importance of childcare and maternal love, while the Jesuits focused broadly on raising and educating the young. The socio-economic circumstances were changing, and mercantilism flourished. A free-market economy got a start together with a beginning industrialization. People began to concentrate less exclusively on their own community. They became more mobile and thereby acquired more freedom. As family members started to focus more on each other, the previous sociability of the village community or neighbourhood became less important.

The quest for privacy was expressed in architecture as well. Parents and children had separate bedrooms. The affective function, formerly filled by the community, now became the family's role. The closed or nuclear family started more or less at the same time as the functional specialization. Thus, the school partly took the child away from the adult milieu and prepared it for learning. In addition, the family began to concentrate on and specialize in rearing the child, so that it had a better chance as an emotional being. Although the father continued to be the boss, the mother henceforth acquired the responsibility within the home, for the '*pater familias*' worked in the outside world. Sexuality came to be more private and hidden. The *Haven in a Heartless World* that the historian Christopher Lasch praised with such passion and that, according to him, is seriously threatened in our time did not become common property until around the eighteenth century.

The nuclear family defined as the single-family and two-generational family was seen as the nucleus that lived inwardly directed, raising the barrier to the outside world. Special children's literature was created, full of warnings and devoid of sexuality. From here on childhood innocence was to be protected from the adult world. Sleeping together in one bed was unadvisable, chastity and taboos against masturbation were recommended, sexual contact with children and the spontaneous expression of sexuality were discouraged.

In addition, individualism gained more space, mutual feelings replaced the dictates of the circumstances, and 'compassionate marriage' took the place of the marriage of convenience. Partners developed empathy for each other and their children, parents had fewer children, and the families grew smaller. Initially, all of this refers primarily to the middle class. While, on the one hand, more attention, love, and care was given to children and material conditions were improving, on the other hand higher demands were made of the child. Not only did it have to attend school to learn and achieve, but it also had to learn to keep its impulses and bodily functions under control. Mothers were urged to give more exclusive attention to their children, starting by breastfeeding them themselves.

In the eighteenth century the first wave of emancipation found its stride as well. The *femmes savantes*, mockingly known as *Les Précieuses*, resisted the moral demand for breastfeeding that was gradually becoming the norm. These women wanted to develop themselves and lead an intellectual life that conflicted with housekeeping concerns. What had become clear in the interim was that a lack of maternal care could have a disastrous effect on the survival chances of the child. The pedagogues of the Enlightenment began to appeal to the guilt feelings of the mother, just as current psychoanalytic pedagogy appeals to the maternal conscience, in particular.

Ever greater demands were made, but not on the mother alone. The greater indulgence towards the child went hand in hand with more coercion, as mentioned above. This process continued until, in the nineteenth century, strictness and punctuality finally reigned supreme. The physical was burdened more and more with taboos while the boundaries of modesty were stretched even further. For the first time in history, toilet-training starts to play a role. Until then, God's water was left to run freely across God's field, although intrusive methods by which to forcibly control the child's insides had long existed. Louis XIII was given thousands of enemas as a small child. Among the middle class, the use of laxatives and enemas only increased in the nineteenth century. People were heavily preoccupied with everything that went 'in' and came 'out'. It could be 'right' inside or 'wrong', and parents entered into the battle against the evil inside the child's body.

All of the above indicates not only a greater involvement with the raising of young children, but also more interference and intrusion. Fighting masturbation grew into a veritable obsession. Doctors revealed themselves to be dangerous persecutors and cruel oppressors – based entirely on moral grounds, although they claimed to be acting from a medical standpoint. Pedagogy used the most barbaric means on the ground of higher principles. Relevant or not, little boys were constantly threatened that their pecker would be cut off. In the nineteenth and early twentieth centuries, threats of all kinds became standard pedagogical methods for fighting masturbation, at least among the bourgeoisie. In the old days the prohibition of masturbation had never been all that strict: the only opposition existing then was to homosexuality among adults. Now parents reacted with overt threats of castration to anything having to do with sexuality. If need be, they would appear with knives and scissors to menace the child who had touched his genitals. Physicians actively interfered: circumcision, clitoridectomy, and infibulation were commonly implemented against the wicked activity. The most ingenious instruments of torture were designed to keep children from masturbating.

Another obsession was that of good posture, with a straight back at all times. Pedagogues never took their eyes off the young, who were no longer in charge of their own body. Around 1850, the apex in physical violence to and moral pressure on the child guilty of transgression had been reached. This violence was now 'scientifically' founded and therefore legitimized, in contrast to the previous impulsive variation. In the eighteenth century sexual contact with children was exposed, in the nineteenth century the child's own sexuality had to pay for it: these measures were inspired by projected personal forbidden desires and yearnings.

Despite the different emotional value the child acquired, many customs that seem ghastly to us today were maintained into the twentieth century. In England small children were still used for going into the narrow, partly flooded coalmine shafts, where they were forced to perform difficult tasks such as raising pulleys and pushing coal-trucks. Furthermore, their working day was closer to 15 than 8 hours in length. The nineteenth-century English novelist Charles Dickens described the fate of children of the industrial period in fine detail. David Copperfield, the protagonist of the novel by the same name, was boarded out at the age of about 11 to work far from home under unspeakable circumstances, without adequate food and without any pay. Poor mothers were wage slaves and were thus unable to take care of their children. At the very time that the greatest material progress was happening, children were still suffering badly.

A few examples will illustrate the distance that separates our contemporary standards from nineteenth-century mores. As a small child in Freiburg where he lived with his parents in one room, Sigmund Freud witnessed the death of his little brother. Gustav Mahler, a contemporary and briefly one of Freud's patients, composed his *Kindertotenlieder* in response to his own experiences as a child. His brothers and sisters died one after another, and later on he even had to live through the death of his own small daughter. It is incomprehensible to us that, after all the neglect and disregard he suffered, the French novelist Honoré de Balzac was able to lead a full life, at least in a creative sense. Compared with children of his time, his life story – sent away as a baby to a wet nurse in the countryside, never visited by his parents, and then sent away to boarding school – was far from exceptional. The breach between Balzac and his mother was never repaired, something that he lamented bitterly. What is extraordinary, however, is that such – in our eyes – terribly 'neglected' children were able to become such sensitive adults, capable of putting themselves inside all kinds of emotional feelings of other people. In other words, this sort of 'neglect' was less exceptional than we would think it to be today. Of course, the writers mentioned here were exceedingly gifted and sensitive by nature. Still, the norm seems to have shifted: what we call neglect and the consequences we attach to it might be strongly linked to specific eras rather than be an absolute concept with eternal value.

Obviously, the relationship between parents and children is a question of social class as well. The bourgeoisie was in the forefront in making demands and paying attention to children, within the framework of the achievement ethic that was part and parcel of the industrial revolution. The norm of the family as breeding ground for the emotions penetrated the working class only slowly, in part because often they were still living in dreadful indigence, certainly up to the First World War.[27]

For example, in north-western Europe around the First World War, well into the modern era, almost half of all the children born were still dying very young, even if abandoning them as foundlings had become a rarity. All forms of neglect, malnutrition, lack of hygiene, and infectious diseases were the cause. Nevertheless, the mentality where children were concerned had gradually changed across all levels of society.

The greatest catalyst of this changed mentality was the introduction of the school and of compulsory education. Schools became an important institution for exercising state control on education and transfer of knowledge. Furthermore, schools removed children from the labour market, which encouraged an emotional appreciation of children who thus grew into emotionally appreciated beings instead of breadwinners.

In the description of previous customs concerning children, one must remember that no connection whatsoever was made between childhood experiences and the later development of the adult. No correlation was made between oppression, powerlessness, and pent-up rage. It was not known that cruelty can be engendered by what one has suffered as a child and that inadequate care and love in the first years of life might result in masochism.

That sadism and masochism tend to appear as a pair, later known as sado-masochism, was not yet known. The history of individual development did not become charted territory until psychoanalysis entered the stage. Empathy with children is a recent idea, while every period, including ours, contains remnants of preceding eras; the life of the musical child prodigy and the athletic child champion are, in a sense, anachronisms that evoke earlier times.

From the eighteenth century onward maternal love was turned into a problem. It became a concept, and thereby a conflict was created between the interests of the mother and those of the child. Initially, in this period there was no question yet either of exclusivity of the mother–child relationship. On the contrary, childcare was still left to the household staff, which only the very poorest could not afford. Sigmund Freud's parents, who, as we saw before, were poor and at first lived in one room with the whole family, nevertheless had a nanny, as did Fyodor Dostoyevsky, the famous nineteenth-century Russian writer. He and his family, too, lived in poverty in Baden-Baden, near a casino. Because he was addicted to gambling, he was penniless for a very long time.

Maternal love after 1900, since Sigmund Freud

Although the classification by round numbers and centuries is an arbitrary one, it can be posited that it was after 1900 that the specific interest in children got started, consisting of thinking about children from the point of view of childhood experiences and not exclusively from the adult perspective. At the end of the nineteenth century the interest in childhood experiences did not go much beyond catching them at and keeping them from forbidden sexuality. Even Sigmund Freud, as a child of his time, was in the beginning still convinced of the harmful influence of masturbation.[28] Nevertheless, he discovered for the first time that the child partakes of infantile sexuality and its accompanying fantasy life.

Initially, the mother is barely mentioned in psychoanalysis. Everything revolves around the symbolic father, who presumably prohibits the little boy's desired relationship with the mother: the Oedipus complex. Melanie Klein, the psychoanalyst of Viennese origin who from the 1920s on lived in London, where she became famous, would later question Freud on this point by emphasizing the prime importance of the bond with the mother. She pays a great deal of attention to the very earliest developments of the child and its inner fantasy world.

Early in the twentieth century Freud describes the treatment of a little boy who suffers from oedipal anxieties and develops a horse phobia: the case history of Little Hans.[29] Among other things, Freud here recounts the castration threat by the mother and the information that Hans requested from his parents but never received. He was preoccupied with the relationship between his parents and the mystery of procreation. This case study is still a fascinating account of a treatment that reads like a novel.

At present we would be less inclined to ascribe Hans' problems mainly to his inner drive development. Greater emphasis would be placed on Hans' emotional bonds, especially the relationship with his mother: the parents' marriage was unhappy, leading to the mother's need for the love of her son that is expressed by her tendency to take him into her bed. In Freud's description, resolving the clearly ambivalent bond with the mother seems to be only a by-product of the treatment. Freud saw mother–son relationships as ideal, excluding any ambivalence. His emphasis was on the ambivalent relationship of the son towards the father. In this case, Hans' father treated his own son, consulting with Freud on a regular basis. This way he gave extra attention to Hans, thereby helping the child to shift the emotional emphasis from mother to father. He thus became less dependent on his mother. But there is no mention yet of the importance of maternal love, materialized in mother's constant care for her child. Neither does Freud say a word about the mother in the Schreber case, nor does it play a role of any importance in the treatment of his patients the Wolf Man, the Rat Man, or Dora.[30]

Since the Second World War, household staff has become a thing of the past. Families have grown smaller and more isolated from next of kin, especially in big cities. Divorce, and fatherless and single-parent families, have become more common. The place of the mother in the young child's life is more central than ever before, as she is often alone with her (young) child. The place of the mother in the child's life, as psychoanalysis sees it, has also changed. The child's fortunes are more specifically connected to emotional interaction with parents, especially the mother.

In the last fifty years the importance of developing a close bond with the mother has been firmly accentuated. Unfortunately, this bond may have a one-sided influence on the child. It increases the danger of a symbiotic, parasitic relationship. The mother becomes the all-encompassing factor, even when due to her own problems her influence is less beneficial. The English psychoanalyst Estela Welldon even speaks of the mother's perverse omnipotence.[31] Growing up alone with a less-than-healthy mother may have consequences that are as serious as those of neglect. However, the solution also does not lie in having the child raised by people other than the parents. Once that was the guiding philosophy behind the Israeli kibbutz: a collective education would lead to the prevention of the Oedipus complex. Later on it turned out that the kibbutz children had actually missed the intimacy with their parents. It was replaced by the proximity of other children, which taught them more about how to be intimate with contemporaries than with one's own partner – for, after all, the relationship with the latter is based on the early experiences with parents. Every era and every ideal creates its own problems. The same is true for the ideal of maternal love, because, obviously, the ideal parent and the ideal education do not exist.

The historian Philippe Ariès correctly points out that the conscious empathy of the modern individual with the small child could possibly conceal an unconscious hatred.[32] In psychoanalysis this is known as reaction-formation: it means that an exaggerated concern can cover up the reverse. Currently, the mother–child relationship is greatly idealized, whereby a symbiotic illusion threatens to be created. On the other hand, with two working parents who are always in a rush, ever-growing emotional neglect is imminent. After the preceding it may seem unexpected, but all the consulted authors agree that, when all is said and done, we are living in a period that is less child-oriented than we might think at first glance. They speak of a crisis in motherhood because maternal devotion is at issue. We have reached a phase in history in which the bond between partners is more central than ever before. The free choice of a partner, the sexual revolution, the lesser parental authority over adolescents, all make partners seek their refuge with each other more than before and less with the children they might have.

Maternal love and symbiosis

Maternal love as an ideal should serve to encourage the development of healthy children. In the past hundred years, after Sigmund Freud, heredity as the cause of disorders was replaced by psychological traumas. Freud himself evolved and often changed his theory. First he blamed pathology on seduction of the small child by a sexually rapacious adult. Later, when he discovered more about individual fantasy life, the child's sexual development and accompanying fantasies were held responsible. Next, after Anna Freud, the mother was considered the central person for the child, just as in the eighteenth century. The theory about the cause of emotional harmony versus psychological suffering thus continues to develop.

The farther back we go into history, the less the opinions about, and the practice of, education are in keeping with our own. Sacrificial maternal love is not a matter of course. Although our present-day ideas about the love and care that children need to become healthy adults seem self-evident to us, these reflections are of rather recent date. Since prosperity creates sufficient room for maternal love, this ideal has become a moral requirement.

The fact that post-war psychoanalysis began to highlight the mother so strongly appealed urgently to her conscience and sense of responsibility. Since mothers have become more aware of the child's need for her love, the ambivalence and hostility towards the child has to be pushed aside. A conflict has emerged insofar as the child's interests do not move in a parallel direction with the mother's. Mothers of young children are often depressed, locked in, and frustrated in their desire to participate in life outside the family. Does this mean that mothers today have become less loving, as the historian Christopher Lasch[33] assumes, based on the increase in early disorders and narcissistic problems?

In more recent decades, pathology of the most divergent kinds is often – and perhaps not wrongly so – attributed to the earliest mother–child relationship. The 'rapprochement sub-phase' of the symbiotic period, in particular, when the child experiments with distance and proximity, involving the mother's attitude towards separation, is considered important.

The danger in searching for the 'causes' of psychic suffering in lack of maternal love is not only one-sided, it also confuses quantity and quality. Fathers are all too often still excluded from consideration, and mothers – not unjustifiably – rebel against the appeal to their conscience and the exclusive responsibility placed upon them. No matter how ideal maternal love may be, it is an illusion to think that the ideal of psychological health will thereby have been attained.

In the welfare state higher demands are made of the affective life, and thus of education that is to lead to 'happiness' through the fulfilment of desires. Our requirements concerning well-being have increased mightily, and our expectations of psychiatry are exaggerated since in the Western world almost all problems are labelled as psychological suffering. Happiness, the goal, is as indefinable as mental health, which is its condition. Maternal love seems more readily definable: the mother simply needs to be there all the time to provide her child with love, which is her task and assignment in life. The supposition is that, as a result, her child will not only be psychologically healthy, but happy as well. This promise is not kept any more than was the promise of heaven in earlier times. Mental health is as rare as a perfect set of teeth: imperfection is the norm.

Today, mothers tend to be better educated and informed than was the case with their parents. This has made their maternal tasks more demanding, not only because in addition to their motherhood they are often socially active, but also because there are no nannies or grandmas who lend a hand any longer, while the father is still absent most of the time. Few mothers are the ideal mother needed to perform such an arduous and difficult task.

Depending on one person only for all affective needs can be agonizing and unhealthy, not only for the mother but for the child as well. Serious pathology, emotional suffering that goes beyond mere neurotic complaints, has lately increased instead of diminished. The 'bliss' of the early mother–child symbiosis is more of an idealization than one that represents reality.

Normally the mother's need for the child is not equivalent to the child's need for its mother. A two-sided symbiosis points to a burdensome parasitic relationship that develops when a mother needs her child to maintain her psychic equilibrium.

Nowadays mothers deem themselves obliged to actualize the idyll of the blissful mother with her child within the family, and they feel they are failing when that does not quite work. We are gradually discovering that maternal love is not the only form of love but that paternal love, too, exists from the very first moment on and is an equally vital bond.[34] When the parental task is shared between two individuals, each with their own contribution to make and their own 'masculine' or 'feminine' approach, the child benefits from the difference in male and female style and the difference in the father and the mother's character. This stimulates its mental development.

The father's role is in the process of changing, and psychoanalysis is paying more attention these days to the father, not as universal symbol of the oedipal father but as a concrete factor within the family. All too often it is unequivocally accepted that everything has to do with the mother where the young – or not so young – child is concerned.[35]

Maternal love put into perspective

We are more anxious than ever before about the quality of maternal love and its continuity, especially during the early years of life. We are discovering gradually that early disorders appear far more often than we used to think, and we interpret that as a lack of maternal love in our harried and materialistic era. At the same time, there is a heavy emphasis on the mother's obligations. In any event, history helps us to put things into perspective.

At present we would describe those patients whom Freud saw and characterized as neurotic, or at most as oedipal, more as borderline, narcissistic, or otherwise suffering from a very early disorder. This may lead us to various conclusions. It remains questionable whether early disorders actually appear more frequently than they did in bygone days. In my opinion, it is more a matter of our having learned to observe better and make more subtle diagnoses. We know a great deal more about children, toddlers, and even babies, thanks to the contributions of psychoanalysis, systematic observation of children, and – the newest shoot on the trunk of psychoanalytically oriented child care – baby and infant research.

Little by little it is becoming clearer that every function and relationship develops much sooner than classical psychoanalysis used to assume. In that respect, Melanie Klein, the psychoanalyst who partly complemented and partly refuted Sigmund Freud's ideas, has been put in the right. The greater attention given to more subtle nuances in the life of the emotions is due to our socio-economic and psychological phase in the 'civilization process', also known as modernization.

The Western world is more prosperous than was ever the case for larger groups in any preceding historical period. Working by the sweat of one's brow has changed into fretting over the strength of our relationships. The demands of modern partner relationships are so high that only affectively satisfied children will be able to fulfil them at all in their adult lives. Expansion of knowledge has both helped and cast a gloom over us. It comes as a profound shock to us that maternal love is not self-evident, as can be clearly seen in video films made during research on interactions between the average mother and her child.

We are much more aware than was previously the case of how dependent we are on the qualities of our earliest caretakers. Sigmund Freud's mother was still able to leave her children in the hands of a nanny without worrying. Too often mothers are forced to take care of their children by themselves today while, at the same time, there are more possibilities for women to develop themselves and participate in the working world. The woman's wider participation in the life of society is a cause for concern for the specialist who wants to see that the young child's potentials for attachment are protected. On the other hand, it may not be all that ideal for mother and child always to be together. An anxious mother may well use her children to fulfil her own unsatisfied needs for love and insist on tokens of love from them. In that case, the children learn to fine-tune their emotional lives to the mother's yearnings and fantasies, so that their own development and independent persona are crushed. Donald Winnicott, the celebrated English paediatrician and psychoanalyst, described this as the false self of the as-if personality, who allows his desires to be guided by his need for approval.[36] The desire is then one of fulfilling the mother's desires in order to obtain her love and approval and avoid her (unconscious) hatred.

We may wonder how the common problem known as symbiotic illusion is generated in those cases where a happy medium is not struck. Important here is the historically developed reality. Too often the mother feels alone and thinks that she has to rely on her child, while the child also, is too much alone with its mother. The dyadic twosome that has to satisfy each other's needs of love has landed in a state of isolation. In our time, mothers often have the idea that they must actualize the idyll of the blissful mother and child, like Mary and Jesus. They think they have failed when this does not work so well. But maternal love is not the only form of love. The father is a factor as well: his love is equally indispensable, and from the very first moment on. The triad is the remedy for the one-sided dyad of mother and child that engenders an undesirable lifelong symbiotic illusion.

The father should not be neglected as an important factor in a child's life. His love is equally indispensable, and that from the very first moment on. The triad is the remedy for the one-sided dyad of mother and child that engenders an undesirable lifelong symbiotic illusion. The father, who might be able to lend support to the mother and stand between her and the child so that symbiosis will lead to individuation, is frequently absent in our 'society without a father'.[37] After being the absolute power for centuries, has he during the course of recent history become the excluded third person? Within the family at least, it seems that the matriarchy has replaced the patriarchy.

Chapter 4

Nina

Daughter of a single mother

Nina and her divorced mother live together as a single-parent family, an increasingly common mode of cohabitation. It is our intention to consider the potential consequences of such arrangements, which usually concern single mothers. How does this situation affect the children?

Such children will often feel a greater responsibility for their mothers than when a father is also present and will have a more difficult time breaking away, because the parent will then be left alone. They will find it harder to leave home and become independent. They might become angry less quickly with an already vulnerable parent. Some mothers find it difficult to maintain discipline, especially with adolescent sons.

Single working mothers have a particularly difficult time of it and easily feel inadequate. They have a tendency to be overindulgent out of a sense of guilt. They will spoil their children materially or in other ways and will put up with more than they would really like to do. Single mothers may experience a loss in status or of financial means that makes raising children extra burdensome. When adversity strikes, single parents will become unsettled more easily: they can expect support only from their child. When depression sets in, the child is alone in taking care of the mother. In short, single parenthood is fraught with innumerable problems.

Daughters especially run the risk of becoming the only source of consolation for a desperate and helpless mother. This will make them swallow normal irritations and keep them from articulating any criticism, which may thwart their development, particularly during puberty. The inclination that girls already have to feel solidarity with their mothers will hereby be reinforced. Thus it can occur that the second separation–individuation phase that adolescence provides may slip away from them.[1] The first time that a child becomes more independent is at pre-school age, when it starts kindergarten, for instance. Puberty is a second phase during which children practise freeing themselves from their parents.

Many mothers who raise their children alone – divorcees or widows, for instance – do so quite well and in as healthy a manner as possible. The less emotionally stable, narcissistically vulnerable, or otherwise unbalanced she is, the more difficult it will be for the mother. She will then be more inclined to seek support from her child or use her child as an extension of herself. With a daughter, in particular, there is a chance that a parasitic relationship may surface, because the mother uses her daughter to relive her own life, for example. As we have seen, the relationship can easily grow into a symbiotic illusion.

A third person, in most cases the father, can help to stimulate independence in the child. The parents can keep each other from extremes and undue accentuations. The differing viewpoints of the two parents create room for differentiation and triangulation. Gender and generational differences are much clearer. Without that third person, higher demands are made on the mother's potential for allowing the child its independence. When the child's emotional interests do not hold a sufficiently central position, the child can become the one who must fulfil the parent's fantasies and act as the recipient of her projections.

Nina in therapy

'I've been sick all week, stomach cramps, fever, I'm really not feeling well. My father [who lives abroad] was in Amsterdam with his wife and children, my mother had her boyfriend with her; he was and still is an old friend of my father's too; we'd all been invited by mutual friends of my parents. It was very emotionally demanding and exciting to have it all come together like this.' In this way teenager Nina tries to express her many dilemmas and loyalty conflicts.

Nina came to therapy once a week, due to fierce arguments with her step-mother that would upset her completely for weeks.

She had primarily grown up with her mother. Her parents had divorced when she was about 3 years old. At that time, the family was living in French Guyana, where Nina was born and raised bilingually. As a small child she had suffered from many contagious diseases.

Nina, who calls her parents by their first names, is convinced that she and her mother think and feel the same way, want the same thing – in short, that she is one with her mother, as it were. In her behaviour Nina comes across as extremely mature. The relationship with her mother often appears to be enacted on a quasi-equal level; mother and daughter behave rather like gen-erational contemporaries.

Nina thinks she knows that she is the most important person for her mother. She can uphold this conviction as long as it suits the latter not to spoil that illusion. When the mother is in love, a regular occurrence, or involved in a relationship, Nina feels slighted. She may become intensely jealous and do anything to play them off against each other.

The relationship between mother and daughter is frequently painful and turbulent, every time the illusion of being-one together is cruelly disrupted.

When peace reigns, when mother and daughter are in agreement, it confirms their unconsciously shared idyll. The mother would regularly confide her problems to Nina from the time that her daughter was very young, and the girl would often have to console her weeping mother. Conversely, the mother used her parental authority to deter Nina from relationships with others. On the one hand, Nina is regarded as an adult, an equal, while, on the other, she is treated as a little child incapable of being responsible for her own comings and goings. In any case, Nina experiences her mother as highly demanding and wanting to be in control of everything. What she does and does not do, whom she sees, what she shares with others, all of it is constantly criticized. In her mind, Nina is kept on a short leash, raised strictly, and had better spend a great deal of time on her homework and other tasks. It seems that mother and daughter keep a sharp and envious eye on each other's potential contacts with any third parties.

To my surprise, after some time it turns out that there is a previously unmentioned third party involved. Nina's mother now has a steady boy-friend, who has also moved in with her. Until now, Nina has kept this man out of our conversations, just as she attempts to keep him out of her relation-ship with her mother as an undesirable third party. While her desire for an idyllic twosome becomes more and more obvious, we can address her anger and sadness about her feeling of being excluded. In spite of her jealousy of her mother's friend, in the end Nina succeeds in developing a bond of her own with this man. In addition to her anger with him, a stepfather–daughter relationship begins to grow between them. Later it will become apparent that the mother tolerates only quite badly this intrusion on the dyad with her daughter; she also has a hard time reconciling herself to the boyfriends that Nina has outside her home life.

Nina fears to disturb our twosome and temporarily avoids telling me with whom she spent the summer holidays. I find out after the fact that Nina had gone camping with two girlfriends during the summer vacation. However, she was utterly miserable because of the intimacy between the other two. As a third party, she felt excluded from this female dyad as well, something not at all unusual among girls.

After two-and-a-half years of treatment, Nina reveals that she now has a close girlfriend, something she never emphasized before. I wonder aloud whether she might fear that I will become envious of her friend. This girl seems more like Nina's shadow than a real person, Nina being mainly pre-occupied with herself and her mother. It strikes me repeatedly how little the people in her daily life come to life as individuals in her story, although Nina is a vivacious young girl and a good talker. Her preoccupation with others or lack thereof is strongly coloured by her frustrations, her sense of being rejected or excluded. She, in turn, is quite capable of excluding whom or what does not suit her.

When the above-mentioned girlfriend unexpectedly loses her father, Nina shows no sign of empathy or compassion. Does her envy of the girl's having had a father nearby while she had to do without one play a role in this? Or are all fathers excluded from the mother–daughter dyad? Do third parties virtually not matter at all, because they only give rise to jealousy? In any event, her reaction reinforces my impression that her inner fantasy life is still dyadically structured. In symbiotic relationships quasi-intimacy and the illusion of complete mutual understanding eliminate an exploration of the other and of any true intimacy. Besides, the several dyadic relationships are kept securely separate, so that a great deal has to be kept secret and concealed. Nina and her girlfriend, Nina and her mother, Nina and her therapist exist side by side as an equal number of illusory dyads that are kept separated.

On the one hand, Nina admires her mother, a talented and creative painter, and likes to be in her proximity. On the other, she constantly deplores the lack of distance between them. She admits how she sleeps in her mother's bed, sometimes for a whole week. She will then fall asleep immediately, in contrast to other times when she is by herself. Undoubtedly it is very flattering and seductive for her when her mother confides in her as an adult, and extremely irritating and taunting when she is excluded from her mother's bed and love life once again. Nina has a weak sense of self-worth and feels inferior with regard to her mother. She sees herself not so much as the beloved one and only child, the centre of her mother's attention, but, rather, as her indispensable extension. The latter forms a painful blow to her narcissism.

At school she is an excellent student who applies herself to her work with great devotion. The results are, indeed, outstanding, but for Nina they are never good enough. Mother is exceedingly ambitious concerning her daughter's accomplishments. In this regard, too, Nina tries to please her mother in every way. Nina is strict with herself: she is chronically exhausted because she goes to bed late as a result of her studies. It all bears out that Nina has incorporated the high demands from both parents into her stern conscience. Moreover, Nina complains that her mother never praises her for her achievements but always thinks she could do better. According to Nina, she also constantly finds fault with her daughter's behaviour as well as her character. Clearly, Nina yearns for love, praise, and affection. She tries to gain extra attention from me and to make me into an ally by telling me how hard it is for her at home.

Where boyfriends are concerned, she will sometimes demonstrate that she feels superior to a boy and looks down on him. At other times she has an intense longing for a specific boy whom she admires and thinks she can never have. Her mother usually disapproves of her choice, and then Nina suddenly loses all interest in him, too. All the same, she will quietly 'go with' a certain boy for a while. Neither her mother nor I will know anything about this. It is the same story all over again: keeping things secret for fear of arousing envy when a third party is involved. She makes love with him, as she later recounts, because she is afraid he will lose interest in her. In other words, even after the fact she will deny to me that she feels anything for another person.

Nina prefers to tell me that she finds little pleasure in her relationships with boys. I suggest once again that she is afraid of making me jealous and therefore she denies finding pleasure in being with anyone else.

She likes to stir things up between people to prevent those two from building something that excludes her. She wants to prove her preference vis-à-vis her mother and me alternately, and she loves to play us off against each other that way. Thus she always has a special little tête-a-tête with each of us separately. She states quite honestly and openly that she always hopes the relationships of her key figures will fail. Like so many children of divorced parents, she has loyalty conflicts. This way, she stood between her father and her mother after their divorce and afterwards between her father and his second wife as well. Initially she tried to create a link with both her father and her stepmother and play them off against each other. It did not work, so she herself became the third party in the game, whereupon she picked a fight with her stepmother. When her father did not take her side but his wife's instead and – in Nina's mind – the stepmother rejected her, she became desperate, which was the reason she started treatment with me.

In her fantasy, Nina's father functions primarily as the excluded third party. Her mother sued for the divorce, while mother and daughter agree in their opinion of him. Nina has rejected her father's family name and has adopted her mother's out of unconscious feelings of revenge against her father and in collusion with her mother. Nina eliminates her father, and yet does not, from her inner world. She keeps double books, as it were. Because of the divorce, she feels disappointed in him, and because of the new marriage, she feels excluded. Not only is Nina consumed with jealousy of her father's second wife, but she is also convinced that the children from this second marriage are much more indulged than she ever was.

How Nina confronts and manipulates her therapist

Nina is charming, not to mention seductive. For a long time, she pretends to be always cheerful and enters my consultation room laughing and talking loudly. She will only gradually show that she feels critically observed and not at all at ease. She is insecure and tries hard to have me like her. Her comings and goings are mostly determined by the alleged wishes of some other.

In addition to a good head for study, Nina also possesses a fine radar where her emotional intelligence is concerned. Yet, although the treatment process is running smoothly, she complains that nothing is happening. Besides, she thinks I do not love and appreciate her. The opposite is true: I always enjoy seeing her and work with her gladly and intensively. She has an excellent ability for following and profiting from my remarks. Between sessions she reflects on herself introspectively. At a subsequent session she usually comes back to what had been discussed the previous time. She definitely understands the effects that interruptions or vacations have on her – they are separations, after all, which she handles badly. In the face of my attempts to discuss our interaction in the transference, her initial disbelief routinely ends up in a newly gained insight. Fortunately, Nina associates easily, and with new associations she proves that she has understood what is going on.

As mentioned above, Nina is sweet and flattering towards me and for a long time hid her despondency and disappointment about the fact that she does not feel appreciated. Gradually, however, the contrary appears: I am nothing but critical towards her, just like her mother. She reacts vehemently to those occasions when I am not there. Although she always acts cheerful and is quick to laugh, she feels greatly wronged. She says that she is nothing but a number to me, one of the many, instead of the only one and the most important one in my life. 'It all means so much to me and so little to you.' She cannot stand that, it makes her angry and desperate. Apparently, she cannot bring herself to the realization that she means something to someone when she is not certain of being the sweetest and the unique one.

To salvage her sense of self-worth, rejection then replaces loving. For Nina it has to be all or nothing. She cannot accept that two people may share something from which she is excluded. Due to the separation of her parents, triangulation has failed. If she is not the only one, she does not count at all. Thus, anything that can divert my attention from her renders her insecure and envious.

From the moment Nina came to me she complained about her mother for a whole year, while I as her therapist remained totally out of range. Hence, she created a split at first, dividing her positive and negative feelings between her mother and me. I am the good object and the mother is the evildoer. Little by little, she is more and more able to recognize the negative, less flattering thoughts concerning me as her therapist.

Progressively she begins to understand her own role: how she provokes her mother to keep her small and subsequently to grow extremely angry about that; how she needs these conflicts and feels lonely and neglected when this interaction does not occur.

She discovers that she has a hard time doing without coercion, and during the transference she repeatedly wants to force me to coerce her. Then I am supposed to give her 'good advice' – in matters of boys, for example. In other words, I have to decide what is best for her, and she grows angry and coercive if I do not do so.

Nina's experience of her relationship with her mother is reflected in the transference, although for a long time she will keep her feelings regarding me to herself. She thinks she is worthless and an extension, unloved and unappreciated. Nina is always tense and afraid of not being liked. For two years she articulated her admiration of me and carefully kept her aggrieved self under wraps. We discover that Nina is envious of me and that in addition to rivalry, she also feels criticism and anger. Thus, she begrudges me the fact that I say something that is helpful to her, or that I might even be right. When questioned, she admits that she is disgruntled because, according to her, I 'never say anything'. She heartily agrees when I verbalize her thoughts as follows: 'What am I actually doing for her, in what way am I helping her at all, what difference does it make to her?' Besides: 'What expertise do I really have?' considering that 'my remarks are never very spectacular, after all'. None of my contributions is of any real consequence. She wants to attack my sense of self-worth, but I almost have to put the words for this into her mouth. Only in a dialogue interlaced with humour does she dare to admit to these thoughts, which reflect her basic attitude.

It is not only Nina's relationship with me that reflects her position to her mother. It is equally recognizable in her relationships with boys. Usually she achieves a role reversal, where Nina is at the centre. The boy has to admire her and be an extension of herself. Her sense of self must be reinforced by his adoration, just as in her own eyes she must reinforce her mother's sense of self-worth. Once the reverse happened: there was a cute boy who would not even look at her. She felt worthless, unattractive, and absolutely miserable. In her eyes, partners are never equals, as one of the two always looks down on the other.

Nina says goodbye

Finally, by mutual agreement, Nina decides to terminate her treatment. I express my suspicion that 'leaving home' will be difficult for her and that she should use this as practice. Terminating therapy will thus become a dress rehearsal, to prepare her for the separation from her mother (the inner one, in particular).

Nina's problematic nature is illustrated by the tempestuous course the final phase of her treatment takes. As usual, with termination all the problems return, though in a nutshell. The reversal, when what has been sown can be harvested and she will admit it has helped her, will not come until the very end. Meanwhile we keep discussing her conflicts in depth without reaching a pseudo-resolution too precipitously.

A central theme is underestimation: her mother feels underrated and unloved by her daughter. Nina, in turn, feels underrated by her mother and her therapist. Nina refuses to recognize the value of the treatment. Out of her anger and disappointment that I can manage without her, she declares the entire venture to have been worthless. By contrast, her sense of not being able to manage without me suddenly grows stronger, which leads her to feel that, once again, she is the vulnerable and inferior party. 'Mirror, mirror on the wall, who is the fairest of them all' remains a weak point in her psychic make-up.

The problems around feeling underrated go back, among other things, to disappointment in her father. She sees him regularly, visits him abroad, and he often comes to the Netherlands. He phones her frequently, and they maintain a regular correspondence. Nevertheless, she has the feeling that she does not really want to know anything about him or have anything to do with him, since he 'abandoned' her. Or is this merely pretence, to keep me happy because, from her perspective, I cannot stand her having a more intimate bond with her father than with me, or with her mother, whose place I occupy in the transference? She underestimates the fact that her father loves her, and she is unable to appreciate what he does for her despite the divorce. This, then, leads to guilt feelings towards him, too.

The painful emotions around the divorce and being left alone with her mother are significantly highlighted again. She is sad that she did not have two parents to raise her together. Furthermore, it put the full burden of the one parent on her and caused the bond with her often depressed mother to become oppressive.

Everything Nina experiences in intimacy with a third party is felt as disloyalty to the mother and/or to her therapist. On the other hand, the mother figure is seen as intrusive. This leads Nina to keep secrets and have trouble with intimacy, with actively sharing what she feels. Her inability to discuss sexuality is one of its manifestations. Still, towards the end she feels freer to talk with me about sex. Nina tells me for the first time that she used to masturbate until she was 11 years old. Thereafter she found it uninteresting and even had an aversion to sex, which grew stronger since she had a sexual relationship at around the age of 14 or 15, while in treatment, which she had concealed from me.

I am utterly astonished to hear this only after the event. The affair developed with the previously mentioned boyfriend, who, she always claimed, was revolting to her. Possibly she only suggests this to reassure me, but she does fear she could have been infected with AIDS and frequently visits clinics to pursue this. Her fear is quite obsessional and might reflect her anxiety around the termination of treatment – as if she wants to let me know that I cannot protect her from this either once she is gone.

Nina has been unable to enjoy a carefree adolescence. She can only sparsely participate in the game between boys and girls. We discuss her problems around boys and crushes. These problems might exist because of her conflicting loyalties, pulling her in two directions. She refuses to do anything that could lead to spoiling the symbiotic illusion with her mother. She would feel guilty about her 'disloyalty' to her mother and her therapist, respectively. Her feelings of loyalty to her father and mother are correspondingly always playing tricks on her. Moreover, giving up the symbiosis would create fear in her of no longer being the most important one for the primary love object. She is married to her mother, as it were, whereby in her fantasy – I carefully presume – she sometimes is the man who is often lacking in her mother's life. Nina confirms this. Furthermore, in a kind of homo-erotic collusion with her mother, men are reduced to worthless 'simpletons' who cannot come within miles of what she and her mother share together.

Briefly, Nina is wholly back in the place where she does nothing but complain about her mother. In an abbreviated form, every symptom will pass in review one more time, as is common in the final phase of a treatment. Additional vicissitudes of the termination phase are illustrative thereof.

During the interruption for my spring vacation Nina falls in love for a short time and is sad when she returns, because the boy has broken off with her. It is both remarkable and unusual because so far she has always been the one who had grown tired of a given boy. Nina understands my comments about feelings of abandonment and how these can shift in her. I suggest that through her crush she has already experienced the end with me and the sense of being abandoned. Losing her boyfriend represents her sense that her therapist has broken off with her. Thus I connect her sadness with having to do without her therapist and the mourning period for which she is preparing.

Nina would always talk non-stop and had also been extremely entertaining as she did so. Now there can be long periods of silence: we are both daydreaming a bit, an atmosphere that has never occurred before. Might she be silently making space in her mind for a benevolent therapist rather than banishing me from her inner life, as she used to do with 'lost love objects' such as her father?

Nina was to play me out one more time, this time against the guidance counsellor of her school, who phones me anxiously: 'If you no longer want to help her, would you be so kind as to refer her for further treatment? After all, the treatment has not helped her at all, she is very unhappy and desperately needs to talk to someone', and so on.

When I see through it as a form of communication by the pulling of strings, Nina can see that she wants to make me pay for terminating. By complaining about me to a third person, she is trying to make a fool of me. She feels caught in the act by me and is quite ashamed of it now. Her role as a schemer who then feels remorse and becomes deeply depressed becomes clear to her. She maligns me in the eyes of others so she will not have to miss me and to deny how much she cares about me, for those are nothing but painful emotions to her.

It is during this final phase of the treatment that I see Nina genuinely sad for the first time. She articulates that she herself wanted to leave because, on the one hand, she wanted to be grown-up; yet, on the other, she regrets it because she feels small and wants to stay with me.

It is remarkable, in the meantime, how well she can acknowledge her feelings towards the therapist that arise in the transference. She no longer circumvents me by complaining about her mother. Just as in frequent sessions of psychotherapy, in once-a-week therapy, too, it is necessary and often possible to deal with transference in order to bring about a process of change.

Nina now sees that she tends to abandon third parties, such as a boyfriend, in order to create a dyad with me that, upon further examination, is a suffocating and illusory one. She understands that she would pay a high price for her illusion around me. Idealizing and admiring me and separating negative feelings means maintaining a quasi-idyllic relationship: that is the way to hold on to me as the only one and to be the only one for me, as is common in the symbiotic illusion, now replaced by a more realistic appraisal of her therapist.

Nina wonders how I will think of her when she is gone. She would so much love to stay and says dreamily how my house, my garden, everything here is so beautiful, so calm. We can now discuss easily that Nina would like us to be 'girlfriends' as a consolation for when the treatment is terminated.

This is followed by a dream in which she is extremely lonely and dies of a dreadful disease. It is reminiscent of her hypochondriacal thoughts about AIDS. Nina quickly comprehends the unconscious connection between departing and dying and recognizes death as a metaphor. Now she is very conscious of the fact that she cares about me, something she had never wanted to admit to herself before. At this point we are dealing with her ability to love. Nina discovers that what she blames me for – lack of interest – is a projection of her own attitude towards others. She articulates her thoughts as follows: 'They're just a number, their stories do not interest me – they're meaningless to me, actually.' What it comes down to is that Nina manipulates people to get her way, just as she herself feels manipulated by the supposed wishes – as she interprets them – of others. Now Nina tells me she is happy that I am the only one who would not be manipulated by her, so that she was confronted with herself again and again, although she was often furious that I would not let her have her own way.

In the interim, Nina has discovered, and to a great extent lost, her own artificiality, her quasi-cheerfulness, her – interest. To her surprise she also discovers she has genuine emotions. She is intensely sorrowful about the farewell, which she compares to dying. Her expressed fear of not being able to handle it all by herself is in obvious contradiction with her previous feeling that I never said anything, never did anything for her, felt nothing for her, and that she would not miss me at all. Now Nina also has a better understanding of why she has always silently accused her parents of not loving her. She now understands that they obviously did love her. It is her own insecurity that causes her to think that others do not like or love her. She realizes that she often yearns for her father. Up to this point she would always describe her correspondence and dinners with him as annoying, routine events, which now changes. Nina appears ready to give greater credit to her father for his loyal attempts to keep in touch with her as much as the circumstances allowed. Now she even states how fearful she is that he might die before she can show him how much she loves him. It seems that her ability for triangulation, for experiencing two parents instead of one, has been strengthened. In the final phase the determinants of Nina's mood are grief over the father, as well as grief over the lost dyad with the mother. She illustrates this through her grief over her cat who has run away. She misses him, especially at night to cuddle with in bed. Then Nina also verbalizes the fear she feels about the future when she will not have me any more.

During the penultimate session Nina recounts that she has been promoted to the highest grade, whereupon she plans to attend university and leave home. She complains to me one last time: she is disappointed in her mother's reaction. All the latter can say is: 'Great that you're on vacation now.' The praise and physical affection that Nina craves so much are not forthcoming. She would not mind being hugged every now and then, she says reproachfully. Yet she fully understands her need to blame her mother for being 'abandoned' by me. She grows calmer when we see the connection between her difficulty with the departure and her complaints about her mother instead of about me for letting her go. Nina is growing more aware of her sense of loneliness. She realizes that she is someone who always longs for love and affection. At the same time she is inclined to distance herself more from complaining about her mother and, after almost three years of therapy, she is more willing to look at herself.

Nina and the symbiotic mother–daughter relationship

This case description illustrates that a symbiosis can be interpreted as a pathological two-sided illusion that can hold a daughter imprisoned. It seems a more fruitful use of the concept than symbiosis as a normal developmental phase. In the latter sense the concept of symbiosis is a controversial topic today. This could lead to considering the concept as antiquated and abandoning it altogether, while it actually can no longer be dropped from the pathology at all.

In my opinion, the concept of symbiosis in its literal meaning is an excellent metaphor for the two-as-one-together relationships described. The mutual dependency in the symbiotic relationship creates an oppressive pseudo-idyll. The lack of separation and the curtailment it causes produce an increase in aggression that is, to a great extent, bound to remain unconscious. The illusion is kept alive, among others, by isolating the hostile emotions and projecting them onto a third person, often the father.

By separating both the object and the self into 'good' and 'bad', the positive relationship with the idealized participant–object can be maintained. Thus the illusion can lead a separate existence, alternating with a consciously felt anger, which was not absent in Nina either.

The dyadic bond of love manifests itself in the need to be the most loved and only one, and in the impossibility of competing with a third person. The existence of that third party is denied in a mutual conspiracy. Every time the illusion is unexpectedly disrupted, the rejection is followed by anger and sorrow.

Nina's symbiotic illusion with her mother served primarily to hide the disappointment in her father, who had disappeared behind an idyll where she believed she did not need him any longer. When she was not able to come between the relationship of the father and stepmother to destroy the new, supremely jealousy-provoking triad, Nina fell into a depression, which led to her treatment.

Because Nina became stuck in, or regressed to, the exclusive bond with her mother, the homosexual object relationship from the earliest phase of life, she has especially intense feelings for various women (just like Dora – see chapter 10): for the mother, the stepmother, one of her mother's women friends, and, finally, in the transference relationship, for me as her therapist. These women are not permitted to know this about each other, for then all hell would break loose. Each must think she is the only one.

The negative transference is kept secret at first in order to suggest and cherish the symbiotic illusion with me as well. Angry feelings do not belong in this illusion and must therefore, by sheer necessity, be lived out via a detour – for instance, by complaining to me about her mother and to her mother about me, while in the meantime keeping the peace with each of us. The dyadic object relationship with her mother is the model for other relationships, both with men and with women. Nina experiences the bond with her mother as coercive and oppressive but also as intensely satisfying.

Obviously, the symbiotic illusion has consequences for the sense of self. Nina's sense of inferiority arises from her position as an extension in the dyad with her mother. This may be a paradox: although she clings to her fantasy of being the only one and thus special, at the same time she is nobody because she has made herself completely dependent. The parasitic party's sense of self-worth is being stimulated at the cost of its 'extension' that, in the end, itself also profits by being indispensable.

Every time the illusion fails to be maintained, the idyll bursts like a balloon, and Nina suddenly and painfully feels herself to be inferior. This leads to the second paradox of the symbiotic illusion. Differences are denied, while the two parts never really become each other's equals. Nina knows just two possibilities: either she is the dependent and rejected one, or she herself looks down on her objects as inferior. What does exist in the symbiotic illusion between parent and child is mutual dependency and lack of differentiation, but there is no equality. The small child is unable to extract itself from the role that its mother has prepared for it. Nina feels that she is a victim while, at the same time, she profits from her position as the indispensable one because that gives her exclusive rights to her mother's love as something that is intended for her alone.

The difference between the generations is usually denied and cancelled. If mother and child are supposedly one and the father is absent, no safe and more stable triangle can be created any more in which generational and gender difference are clear. Girls experience their first love relationship with someone of the same gender. In that sense they are born into a homosexual object relationship, in the erotic sense of the word as well. This first homo-erotic bond will subsequently leave its traces. It is the first crucial phase for the girl before the heterosexual option is added when the father acquires more importance for her. For the boy, heterosexuality in the mother–son relation-ship is a given from the very start. It provides him from the outset with a means by which to distinguish and separate himself. Because for the girl the gender difference is missing as a first incentive in the development towards becoming a separate individual, the temptation is great to linger in the mutual identification that is characteristic of mother and daughter. It does not threaten the girl's sexual identity, as is the case for the boy. However, transfer-ring this love to the man can turn out to be a problematic step, as Sigmund Freud described, stating that a woman often recognizes her mother in her (first) husband.

Nina was a charming and intelligent girl, very attractive, but artificial and quasi-sincere as well. She was bent on seducing her objects into liking and praising her, for her sense of self-worth was extremely fragile. She was not properly rooted in the oedipal triangle and functioned mostly in a dyadic fashion. She always became exceedingly jealous when 'someone who was hers' had shared something with a person other than herself. Conversely, she was also afraid of the jealousy of her key objects when she herself stepped outside the dyad and a third person entered her life. She was fond of intrigues to counteract those situations of which she was fearful.

During the first year of her treatment, Nina was usually in a somewhat excited and overly cheerful mood. She seemed to be taking solace from the illusion that she had succeeded in eliminating her rivals and reserving both her mother and me for herself alone. Nina's agitation would increase at times when this illusion threatened to be disrupted: when her mother was angry with her or when one of her mother's boyfriends seemed to be more import-ant than Nina herself. She was repeatedly desperate – for instance, when her father and stepmother would not allow her to split them apart. Most of the time she did manage to be the only one for her mother who leaned on her and often needed her comfort. Her mother's partners were less threatening because they tended to change, at which point she, together with her mother, could look down on these men. Thus Nina would remain the first, after all, at least in her fantasy, and she would feel less threatened than by her father and his marriage, over which she had no hold. Still, she was always anxious with her mother, too, and busily striving to please her. When Nina felt excluded from her mother's relationship with a man, she would stir up trouble and manipulate to get between them and have her mother to herself again. Never-theless, Nina never felt appreciated and had difficulty appreciating others as well.

Nina was shockingly bad at experiencing reciprocity or at feeling equal to others. There was no question of a true exchange as long as the illusion of a wordless mutual understanding and intuiting was maintained. All this seemed to be the result of a lack of separation from her mother imago. Following a highly classical mother–daughter pattern, Nina thought that if she were to distance herself from her mother, the latter would interpret this as hostility.

Nina's contribution to this struggle for autonomy grew to be workable and negotiable. Finally, Nina gained the insight that she herself, too, had trouble putting her place in her mother's life into perspective.

In the course of her treatment Nina benefited increasingly from our explorations. She was able to verbalize her feelings for her therapist even when they were not flattering – for example, when she would run me down in her thoughts by telling herself that 'it was doing her no good at all', that I 'was worthless', and so on. Then she would feel guilty again about having such thoughts because thereby she was trivializing me and banishing me from her inner world. However, she understood quite clearly that it had to do with the intense humiliation caused by her need for me. And it had to do with a reversal: instead of my having power over her, she made me powerless.

In the end, the termination worked as a new therapeutic impulse that led to a satisfactory resolution after 'repetition and working-through'.

Thanks to the treatment, Nina became less anxious and nervous. In addition, the unprocessed grief from her childhood years became attainable again. She was finally able to grieve over her father's having departed when she was a little girl. She also sensed that she lacked a parent who can step back: one who is clearly from a different generation and with whom she is not locked in a symbiotic illusion, as with her mother. By separating from her therapist, Nina made a start in processing her loneliness and in developing the individuation vis-à-vis her inner mother imago.

Nina had the ability to understand that together we were exploring her psychic reality. She was extremely good at differentiating fantasy from reality, which was a huge help in the treatment of her conflicts.

Chapter 5

Electra versus Oedipus

One might wonder what would have happened had psychoanalysis been the brainchild of a woman rather than of a man. Instead of the Oedipus story – a man's drama – it is likely that the myth of Electra would have been the point of departure. It offers an excellent illustration of some of the pitfalls that women face in their development. Had the first psychoanalytic thinker been female, the mother might well have played a far more significant role. It was not until after he had formulated the greater part of his theory that Freud described the emotional ramifications of the special mother–daughter bond.

In 1931, at the age of 75, Freud admitted in all honesty that the female sphinx continued to be an unsolved mystery to him: 'Nor have I succeeded in seeing my way through any case completely . . .' (p. 227),[1] he wrote. He ultimately confessed that the Oedipus complex was applicable to the development of girls only to a very limited extent.[2] The concept would have to be greatly expanded if it was to pertain to women as well. To preserve 'the core of the neurosis', the Oedipus complex, Freud coined the term *pre-oedipal* and referred to the lengthy pre-oedipal stage in girls. He was therefore well aware of the difference between boys and girls with regard to their development. Nevertheless, he tried to reduce boys and girls to the same denominator of the Oedipus complex. He did so by creating space for the special and protracted mother–daughter bond, thus essentially sidestepping the issue of the Oedipus complex in girls.

I would like to delve more profoundly here into the Electra figure that was introduced in Chapter 1 as paradigm for female development, because this myth attributes a central position to the mother–daughter relationship. Starting at birth, the fate of a woman is shaped by the various aspects of ambivalence towards her mother.

The mother occupies a permanent and central position in the life of every woman. The first love relationship girls have is a homosexual rather than a heterosexual one. After all, their first love object, the mother, is of the same sex. She is also the person with whom the daughter will primarily identify. These two factors combined impose on the daughter a dual loyalty towards her mother. Moreover, irrefutable biological facts make her individuation and sexuality – but not her sexual identity – more conflict-ridden than is the case with boys. Each further step the girl takes in her development must perforce lead to a renewed identification with her mother. This means that with each step forward – like menstruation, initiation into sexuality, pregnancy, giving birth, menopause, and the end of life – she runs the risk of falling back onto her mother or on inner comparisons with her.[3]

'We should expect to see the woman revisiting, re-examining, and resynthesizing representations of self-versus-mother and self-with-mother over a lifetime' (p. 601).[4] There is an ongoing internal dialogue that continues between the two. Does the girl exchange her mother for her father as the most important object? Or does she add a heterosexual object to the given homosexual relationship? Classic psychoanalytic theory on female development presumes the former, but I think there are more grounds for the latter.

In addition, I would also like to pay attention here to the following question: What does women's discontent have to do with the mother–daughter issue? In other words: What is the role of identification, individuation, and separation in female development?

Electra

The character of Electra has always appealed vividly to the imagination. She has been the subject of numerous classic and contemporary works by authors fascinated with the mysteries of the female psyche.[5] Electra represents the problems of less successful female development, in which extreme jealousy, masochism, dramatization, the rejection of femininity, and inhibited sexuality often play a role.

A work of art or a mythological story can be compared to a dream: it is not reality, it is a representation of reality. Symbolic events charged with special significance are vehicles by which to convey various emotions and fantasies. Electra represents the mother–daughter conflict that is laden with fantasies of murder and suicide, with hatred leading to both masochism and sadism alike. Electra is sometimes called hysterical, but the term is then used in the popular derogatory sense of the word because of her assertiveness, her noisy mourning, and her dance of love around her father's corpse, culminating in her delusion of conversing with him.

The myths of Oedipus and Electra are very different in nature, although they both address a child's rivalry with the parent of the same sex and love of the parent of the opposite sex.[6] The guileless Oedipus, woeful son of the king of Thebes, who was almost killed by his own parents, had no intention of murdering his father. He did not even know his father and was fleeing from his alleged parents – actually his foster parents – because of the oracle's prediction that he would kill his father.

For years, Electra was plotting her mother's cold-blooded murder that she would slyly have another person commit. Oedipus, on the other hand, murdered a total stranger on the road to Delphi in an outburst of senseless rage. Electra fostered a lifelong resentment that will become part of her identity once her mother and her mother's lover, Aegisthus, killed Electra's father, Agamemnon, when he returned home in the company of his mistress, Cassandra. After years of waiting and with her brother's help, Electra finally succeeded in taking revenge and murdering her mother, Clytemnestra.

Ancient Greek and modern authors all agree that Electra's rage and loudly bellowed laments are intended as an indictment against her mother, of whom she saw herself, rightly or wrongly, as the unloved victim. It remains difficult to understand why Electra continued to such an extent to idealize her father Agamemnon, the ruthless killer, notwithstanding all the evidence of his selfishness, cruelty, and unfaithfulness. Not only had he murdered Clytemnestra's first husband and children, but he also sacrificed their daughter, Iphigenia, just to appeal to the goddess Artemis for a fair wind. Thereafter he set sail for Troy immediately to go to battle as the Greek commander-in-chief. All this had happened when Electra was still a child. He could not have been much more to her than the myth of an invisible father.

Electra grew up to be an unhappy, lonely woman, obsessed with the acrimony she harboured against her mother and her stepfather, Aegisthus. Demonstrably upset by her admittedly sad fate, she was chronically enraged, deeply disappointed, and weeping loudly for days on end. As she was the potential mother of a male heir to the throne, Aegisthus had banned her from the palace, while their mother exiled her beloved brother, Orestes, to a distant country. As if she had split her feelings into two opposite poles, she hated her mother as much as she loved her father. In his absence, she strongly identified with the father she idolized.

In psychoanalysis this is known as identification after object loss – something we can encounter any day: the bereaved person starts to resemble the deceased. Sometimes, after their mother's death, women begin to identify with her to such an extent that they virtually turn into her. My patient Mira moved into her mother's home, wore her clothes, and defended her in an utterly unreasonable fashion to a sister who dared to criticize the deceased. Annabelle, who had regular conflicts with her authoritarian, demanding mother and was crazy about her father, made a complete turnaround after her mother died. She became furious with her father, would not see him any more, and could not tolerate the slightest criticism of her mother.

Women's stronger bisexuality – wanting to be a man and have a woman while also wanting to be a woman and have a man – is easily recognizable in Electra. Her desire to both be and have a male and a female is expressed through the fact that she disparages her husband (according to Euripides), cuts her hair, and forces her brother to be her implement in the murder of her mother, as if, in her fantasy, she is a man. Her masculinity complex is in evidence when she calls Aegisthus a woman, thinking herself to be more of a man than he is – something that may also attest to her unspoken amorous feelings for her mother and her jealousy of Aegisthus. Her passionate denial of the bond with and the love for her mother are more likely to indicate the repression of the contrary. As Electra's accusation of neglect implies, it is rather a matter of fierce yearning for the love of a nurturing mother and a desire to return to the lost paradise, the close homosexual bond from the earliest part of her life.

The above-mentioned bisexuality may lead to asexuality, as in the case of Electra, who is neither man nor woman and who finds solace in a moral superiority towards her more level-headed sister Chrysothemis, who represents the healthy woman. Electra's anticipation of being the target of her mother's hatred is, in part, a projection of the hostility of the frustrated child. Actually, Clytemnestra is equally as helpless a victim of fate as is Electra, and she, too, has a childlike yearning for a loving mother. Sleepless and consumed by fear, she roams around the palace at night with a sense of guilt as great as that of Lady Macbeth: a female emotion that does not seem to bother most male protagonists and that Electra drowns out with her loud protests. In her despair, Clytemnestra looks to Electra for comfort, almost as if the latter is her mother, and not her daughter. This moment of weakness only arouses contempt and mistrust in Electra, who will seize the opportunity to murder her mother.

From mother to daughter

The God of the Old Testament was known as an envious God who created man in his own image. In real life it is in women's power to produce a human being in their own image, a source of male envy. Not so in the Bible, where God created woman from one of Adam's ribs. She was born as the creation of a 'pregnant' man – just as Pallas Athena was born from the head of Zeus – and was nothing more than an incomplete part of his larger whole.

All this is mythology, while in reality it is woman's fate and destiny to recreate herself in the person of her daughter much more than in that of her son. This is why mothers and daughters are more strongly and more ambivalently attached to one another than are mothers and sons. It is true that a mother's close connection to her daughter can have many advantages, such as teaching her the art of mothering. On the other hand, there is the risk that a lack of maternal love may be passed on by her as well. Generally speaking, the bond between mothers and daughters facilitates passing on emotional health as well as pathology to the next generation via the female line.

Clare

At the age of 25, Clare went into therapy because she had trouble starting a stable relationship with a man. She had an eating disorder, consisting of alternately stuffing herself and vomiting, in much the same way as a patient with anorexia nervosa. She could not have an orgasm without masochistic fantasies. Her aggression took some detours and sometimes took its course via others. One of her boyfriends committed suicide, as did her mother later on.

Clare was in therapy with me for several years, and even long after we were finished she would still come back at moments of crisis or concern. After she completed treatment, she found a suitable husband with whom she bought a house and started a family. She was a good wife and mother, had a part-time job as a physical therapist, and was generally happy with her life.

During the treatment her eating disorder disappeared fairly quickly, but the masochistic fantasies continued. I viewed this as a symptom of an underlying problem related to the struggle she was waging in her mind with her mother. She had the feeling that, unlike her older brother, she was an unwanted child. Her mother had not been happy with her father and had a lover when Clare was a child. As far back as Clare could remember, her mother would disappear at least one day a week and would have long, secretive telephone conversations.

Clare was always afraid of her mother's 'hostile look' and did everything she could to please and placate her by being sweet and obedient. In her fantasies she cultivated the illusion of a tacit understanding with her mother who, in reality, tended to lean on her. In contrast, Clare had hardly any emotional connection with her father, of whom I never gained a clear picture during the treatment.

Clare did not experience puberty, in the sense that she never rebelled. When for the first time she openly exhibited any resistance, she was already in her thirties. Soon afterwards her mother, who was chronically ill at the time, committed suicide. Although her mother had been planning suicide earlier in her life, Clare was tormented by remorse and feelings of guilt.

Whenever she entered my office, Clare always had a frightened expression on her face and would shake my hand stiffly, indicating tension and fear. No matter how hard we worked on her fear of rejection, she remained insecure. She could not bring herself to express any criticism of or hostility towards me. We did not succeed very well in resolving her 'symbiotic illusion' with the therapist and curing her of her split-off hatred. She appeared to be experiencing the therapeutic relationship as a secret idyll from which any hostility had to be banned. I was her guardian angel to whom she sometimes felt closer than to her husband. Concurrent with this internal scenario, she also created a realistic, safe, and trustworthy bond with me. As I saw it, she was managing to isolate her concealed hatred and her feeling of being her mother's victim, turning these against herself via her masochistic sexual fantasies.

It was not until well into the treatment, when we were once again exploring the roots of her uncertainty and fear of rejection, that she revealed a family secret that concerned four generations and went back several generations along the female line. Her great-grandmother worked as a housekeeper, and her daughter – Clare's grandmother – had been born in secret. She was the illegitimate child of the master of the house. To avoid scandal, the biological mother was sent away while the wife adopted the baby to be raised as her own.

It is easy to imagine how much this woman must have hated the daughter whom her adulterous husband had conceived with the servant. The resentment and hatred, which the daughter felt as being directed at her, were of a nature that caused her to leave home as soon as she could. She left for the Dutch East Indies to seek her fortune. Far from home, she found a husband, had some children, and was then divorced again. One of her children was my patient's mother, who sued for divorce from her husband as well. There were times when Clare considered divorce herself, but she never pursued it. Thanks to the insight she acquired in the course of her therapy, she recognized that her own discontent was related to her mother, not to her husband.

Subconsciously Clare was afraid of me. She feared that despite our good working relationship, she was unwelcome and unwanted. Thus, in addition to the symbiotic illusion she maintained, there was another scenario containing these subconscious negative feelings that she inherited from her mother and grandmother.

I realized that Clare was dealing with larger issues than those within her own life experience. These must have been passed on from mother to daughter ever since her great-grandmother was sent away while her daughter became a despised reminder of a humiliating event in the eyes of the adoptive mother. This unfortunate trans-generational mother–daughter conflict illustrates how problems that are pathogenic are passed on via the maternal line. In Clare's case, a fundamental insecurity had been passed on, having started with her great-grandmother.

In Clare I saw evidence of a remarkable coexistence of successful individuation side by side with an unsuccessful separation. She never broke completely free from the conflicts with her mother, but she did manage to keep the conflict largely out of her everyday life. She was a realistic, decisive, well-adjusted woman. In addition, there was a split-off conflict-ridden area that made her yearn for fusion and produced secret fantasies about being a victim and an extension of her mother. She projected these conflicts onto her male partner, which, in turn, led to the previously mentioned sexual problems. The hatred towards her mother, with which she had never come to grips, was now being projected onto the analyst. A repetition of this problem in the succeeding generation of Clare's children could fortunately be prevented. Clare has three happy, successful daughters. It is my experience that therapy can be extremely effective in blocking the transference of problems to the next generation.

Thus, many additional examples can be presented of mothers who continue to play a central role in the life of their daughters.

Elisabeth

A university-educated woman in her late forties, Elisabeth avoids eye contact and, with her dejected appearance, comes across as the embodiment of deep, unspoken sorrow. After years of therapy she surprises me one day with the revelation that as a child her mother had suffered from polio, which had left her severely handicapped. Elisabeth leads a relatively solitary existence. She has had a male friend for years, but he is married, and they only see each other occasionally. Later on she falls in love with a woman – something that had occurred in her adolescence as well. Finally, the two women decide to move in together after Elisabeth had hesitated for a year – she did not want to let go of her man friend, and she did not want to lose her woman friend.

When her weekly sessions are switched to a more frequent analysis, she is still unable or unwilling to tell me even the slightest thing about the physical aspects of either relationship. Sexuality is not discussed: in Elisabeth's discourse, the body is absent. Her problem is that she has an extremely low opinion of herself and is too ashamed to articulate her feelings. Asking for something is absolutely impossible for her, not to mention standing up for herself to obtain what she wants.

Insofar as she can recall, she has always felt that the relationship with her mother was tense and hostile, although neither of them ever acknowledged this openly. Her mother would be waiting for her with the teapot after school. She would praise Elisabeth, approve of everything she did, and on the surface it seemed that all was well, but there was no emotional communication, no real contact. According to Elisabeth, her mother only touched on rather meaningless subjects, which amounted to trivial conversations.

When Elisabeth was about 8 years old, her mother had a 'hysterical' attack, whereby she threw herself on the floor, kicking and screaming: 'I can't take it any more, I won't take it any more!' Elisabeth took revenge by not speaking, vexing her mother with her silence. As long as she can remember, she has wanted to avoid being like her mother in any way possible, while she was crazy about her father, whom she idealized. However, neither parent ever asked her how she was or how she felt. Elisabeth had been a lonely child, which she blamed exclusively on her mother. Her father had worked in a different town and had had little time for the children. It is not until she is in treatment that Elisabeth discovers he never gave her any support or recognition. He did not behave like a father, and he left the care of the house and the four children entirely to the mother, whom everyone therefore considered a courageous woman. She never complained and did not discuss her handicap. Problems were approached exclusively by denial.

In the analysis it becomes clear that Elisabeth identifies strongly with her physically challenged mother, and instead of having physical impediments she feels emotionally handicapped. In the transference she is as uncommunicative with me as previously she used to be with her mother. She is vague, polite, and when she speaks it is in an impersonal, bureaucratic language without emotion. As soon as she is emotionally involved and feels what she recounts, her emotions overwhelm her, and she begins to cry. However, most of the time she is depersonalized, which is to say, she is out of touch with her feelings. This shows in her absentminded moods, which occur frequently: for instance when her purse or her bicycle is stolen, or the time that she left her expensive flute on the train.

Apparently Elisabeth, who has always tried not to resemble her mother, is totally entangled in a repetition compulsion. Unwittingly, she has taken on the burden of her mother's unaccepted handicap. The unprocessed and unexpressed parental traumas by necessity leave communication gaps between parent and child. Parents often tend to conceal shocking things from their children with the idea of wanting to spare the child. However, the result is usually more damaging than the truth would be. Elisabeth has developed a pattern of suffering and denial that is comparable to her mother's. She says nothing but talks cultivated 'nonsense'. In Elisabeth's case the pattern encompasses two generations, for there are no children in whom this emotional blockage can be repeated. In Nora's case, we are dealing with at least three generations.

Nora

This woman, who is in her early forties, came to me because of serious inhibitions in the sexual, professional, and social realm. She feels extremely insecure about her professional status and about her role as lover, wife, and mother. Furthermore, she is concerned about the development of her young daughter, who has once threatened her with a knife. They communicate with difficulty and their relationship is tense. Nora is a devoted but somewhat compulsive mother, who went through an overlooked – neurotic, to be distinguished from psychotic – postnatal depression. Moreover, the baby suffered from serious intestinal cramps and was put on a strict, limited diet for about five years.

Nora feels that her mother is pathologically intrusive and offers innumerable concrete examples of this. Not only does the mother wish to decide how Nora ought to behave but also what she ought to feel. Mother knows better than she herself does what she likes, what she enjoys eating, and what her preferences are. Nora is repelled by her mother and does not dare touch her. Just being in her proximity is torturous for Nora. Consequently, when her own daughter is born, she does not want her mother anywhere nearby. She withholds from her parents the information that she is in analysis. In fact, she never really tells her mother anything about her personal life, and she is constantly anxious about remarks and criticism of the inner voice of her (internalized) mother.

Nora comes from an orthodox Protestant background with strong prejudices against outsiders. Socially conformist behaviour is important to the mother. Nora married a man who fell totally short of her mother's demands. On the other hand, his somewhat crude ways and his sloppy appearance are thoroughly pleasing to Nora. He is everything that, unconsciously obedient to her mother, she may not and dare not be. Her father plays a subservient role in her life. Just like Elisabeth's father, he is a slightly spineless, withdrawn man who, where the children are concerned, leaves everything up to the mother.

Nora has been afraid of her little girl from the moment she was born. She tried to satisfy every one of her child's whims to keep her from crying, for that would make her look like a bad mother. Sometimes she even had the impression it was her critical mother lying in the cradle. At the same time she idolized the baby, while not allowing the hate that was there as well to enter her consciousness. She felt that she, Nora, was bad through and through and that the baby was a perfect and marvellous creature. However, the results were detrimental. In her eyes the child was so exceedingly gifted that she had to learn to read and write even before she could speak properly, and all this while normal communication between mother and child was already blocked. Nora would rarely make little sounds or speak to her baby. The atmosphere between the two was extremely tense.

Nora also idealizes the analyst. She fears my criticism and dreams of assaulting me, without there being any conscious feeling of hatred. Nora has always aspired to being as little like her mother as possible – the Greek tragedian Aeschylus had Electra speak these words: 'And actions and thoughts different from those of my mother, that is my wish.' Nora does not realize that perhaps she is behaving towards her child in the same intrusive, restraining fashion as her mother did, and still does, to her.

To her great relief, contact between Nora and her daughter improves noticeably during the analysis and thereafter, as she tells me much later. The girl becomes more open about her feelings and less defensive with regard to her mother. Although Nora now feels much better about herself and her daughter, the relationship with her own mother remains well nigh unchanged.

Nora demonstrates how pathology is passed on across three generations along the female line. Elisabeth and Nora both had a positive attitude towards their father, but during analysis they each discovered that their relationship with him was far from intimate. Both fathers had kept their distance and were idealized by their daughters, exactly as was the case with Electra. Both women hated their mother and tried desperately not to be like her; identification with her was impeded and curtailed.

They rarely mentioned the body, the representation of the inner mother–object, and experienced it reluctantly. Although the mothers themselves thought their marriage was good and that they were good mothers, the daughters tried to avoid being like them in any way whatsoever; resemblance to their mothers was something of which they were mortally afraid.

There was no sign in either of the two women of an object shift from mother to father. The mothers continued to occupy a central place in the daughters' lives.

Elisabeth's female partner had fine empathy and, in that sense, was different from her mother. Erotically speaking, Elisabeth and Nora were both strongly inhibited, and sexuality was not mentioned, certainly not described in any detail. Neither woman could ever even utter the word penis or dick. The body – their own or that of the other – was taboo, and it remained a subject not to be discussed. The internal mother, her voice, her criticism were persistently feared, and resistance against those was necessary to safeguard their own integrity.

Elisabeth looked rather asexual and neutral where gender was concerned. While she was impeccably dressed, she lacked sex appeal. Nora was more feminine and not without charm, but she felt uncomfortable in her role as lover. She thought she was ugly and dirty and certainly not attractive. Neither Elisabeth nor Nora had succeeded in freeing themselves from their inner mothers.

The problems of Electra and similar women

Sigmund Freud admits that his statement about the Oedipus complex

> applies in complete strictness to the male child only and that we are right in rejecting the term *Electra complex* [Jung's suggestion], which seeks to emphasize the analogy between the attitude of the two sexes. It is only in the male child that we find the fateful combination of love for the one parent and simultaneous hatred for the other as a rival.
>
> (pp. 228–229)[7]

Freud displays his lesser empathy with women here. In my opinion, the Electra complex describes the much more fateful combination in the woman – that is to say, her love for and hatred towards the *same* parent, the mother. It is precisely because of this that girls so often become entangled in ambivalence conflicts. Freud seems to admit here that male and female development does not run analogously. He goes on: 'The turning away from the mother is an exceedingly important step in the development of the girl, it is more than merely an object shift'; somewhat later he repeats: 'The path to femininity development is now open to the girl, insofar as that is not impeded by the remnants of her pre-oedipal attachment to the mother.' Still, the question remains whether a girl can and should overcome her attachment to the mother, as Sigmund Freud believed. Does the consciously rejecting attitude not betray an unconscious attachment to the mother? Furthermore, I suspect that this hostile turning away, as Freud assumed, does not bode well for the development of femininity. As I see it, this indicates unresolved conflicts with the internal mother rather than an object shift.

Apart from the question of whether the girl actually does turn away from her mother, one can expect negative feelings to create a stronger bond than positive ones. Long-lasting hatred of and disappointment in the mother lead to disorders, and these female disorders are mythologically embodied in Electra.

Sigmund Freud and the female Oedipus complex

Sigmund Freud's analysis of Dora,[8] a 17-year-old girl suffering from hysteria (Freud speaks of her as an 18-year-old, but later research proved that she was younger), who came to him at her father's request, generates doubts concerning the Oedipus complex as the cause of her complaints. Rachel Blass writes: 'Freud's move to the classical oedipal model was made possible . . . only by his shifting the focus of theoretical conceptualizations to the analyses of his male patients'.[9]

To be precise, Freud had changed his views in 1897: up to that time he had believed that sexual traumas, such as incest, were the sole cause of neurosis, but thereafter he came to understand that in the creation of all kinds of delusions and misperceptions, the fantasy world, the inner reality, is at least as important as the exterior world.

Freud assumed that Dora's Oedipus complex – namely the strong bond with her father – was the cause of her suffering. She had a negative, ambivalent relationship with her mother and thus was all the more attached to her father. However, he was involved in an affair with the neighbour, Mrs K, which made Dora jealous. She wanted her father's attention, of which she received too little. In turn, the neighbour's husband, Mr K, fell for Dora, which frightened the young girl. His near-assault provoked feelings of revenge in Dora. Her desire was directed not so much at Mr K but at his wife, from whom she sought maternal love.

Dora was presented to Freud by her father, in part because he did not want his relationship with the neighbour to be divulged or impeded.

The treatment was unsuccessful: Freud did not adequately understand the young girl; he was more intent on having his theoretical insights confirmed. Dora resisted and abandoned the treatment after only three months, which Freud attributed to feelings of revenge against men. He was certainly not entirely wrong, and thus the hysterical revenge type was born.

After the Dora debacle Freud did not publish any further case histories by which to corroborate the existence of the Oedipus complex in women. He came to see that his understanding of women fell short, although he could not quite put his finger on it.

Towards the end of his life, Freud returned to the problem of female development. He wrote about the lengthy pre-oedipal relationship of the girl with her mother. At this point, the mother began to play a greater role in his thinking, and the female Oedipus complex was not mentioned again. Before that, he had published a few case studies about women, but those were precisely the cases that did not develop according to the norm of the Oedipus complex. They involved a lesbian and a woman with paranoid delusions, and in both cases it was the mother who was the protagonist in the daughter's mind. Thus, Freud was perfectly aware of the importance of the mother, but he was hampered by his oedipal theory by which the father rather than the mother holds the central position for a girl.

The homosexual girl[10] entered into an erotic connection with a woman after she felt rejected by her mother. For the woman whom he presents in the famous case of paranoia it is the internal mother who determines whether sex with a man is permissible.[11]

The latter reminds me of my patient Nora again, who had the feeling that her mother was lying under her bed whenever she was making love to her husband. Women tell me fairly often that their mother is disturbingly present in the room when they are making love, and mama is also regularly there in a corner of my consulting room.

The lengthiest (unpublished) analysis Sigmund Freud ever conducted with a woman was probably the one of his own daughter Anna.[12] One may assume that her analysis helped him to continue his belief in the female Oedipus complex: Anna was, after all, strongly attached to her father, much more so than to her mother, towards whom she was unfavourably disposed. All of this seems to corroborate the oedipal model, although Anna's development cannot have impressed Freud as being completely feminine.

Freud's opinions on femininity seem to be strongly influenced, nevertheless, by the experiences with his daughter. His article on femininity and that on female sexuality[13] are both highly reminiscent of Anna's analysis, as she herself described it on several occasions. She was a courageous young woman, daring to go into analysis with her father and reveal her secret, rather masculine masturbation fantasies to him. It is with admirable candour that she would later in the correspondence with her closest friends discuss this episode in her life.[14]

In Freud's 'A child is being beaten'[15] – which seems, to a great extent, to have been based on Anna's masochistic problems – girls conceal their oedipal wish behind the unconscious masturbation fantasy that they are being beaten by their father. A daughter's love for and attachment to her mother are here not mentioned more than once. Around 1925, Freud still expressed his opinion that girls hate their mothers;[16] however, nowhere does he mention the possibility that masochism appears in women as the result of the relationship with their mothers.

Later, in 1931, Freud came to the conclusion that women are often unable to overcome their attachment to their mothers. He acknowledged that this discovery was a threat to the Oedipus complex, the cornerstone of his theory, and the 'kernel of neurosis'.[17] Instead of revising his theory and positing the possibility that women have no Oedipus complex, or a different one from men, he formulated the supporting hypothesis of a longer pre-oedipal phase in women. They remain attached to their mothers for a longer period than he had originally thought. When the girl is about 5 years old, she rejects that mother in her disappointment and turns to the father – the reason being that the mother cannot give her a penis, while the father is able to give her a child, at least in the little girl's fantasy world. The object shift that, according to Freud, takes place only later allowed him to restore the Oedipus complex as central paradigm for both boys and girls.

Anna's analysis is likely to have had far-reaching consequences for Freud's view on the supposed object shift in the little girl, 'that destroys the girl's powerful attachment to the mother'.[18] This analysis, this single case, helped him to maintain his theory, at least in part.

Anna, the unwanted last child of the Freud family, felt neglected and deeply disappointed in her mother. She then became extremely attached to her father, whom she idealized, just as Electra did, without attaining a heterosexual object choice in the end. Therefore her development was anything but normative for the development of a woman. She shared her adult life with a woman – the American divorcee and millionaire's daughter Dorothy Tiffany-Burlingham and her four children – and for the rest of her life she remained fascinated with women and mothers.

As in other cases, one might question Freud's premise of a normal object shift. Rejection of the mother and of femininity cannot be termed 'normal' and was, indeed, not so in Anna. As described by herself, her analysis had a great deal to do with renouncing masochistic clitoral masturbation fantasies while the fantasy of being a man also caused her great concern.[19] I fear that Freud's treatment rid his daughter not only of her masochistic fantasies but also of her opportunities for sexual gratification. Her oedipal development, her lack of heterosexual preferences, cannot have made an exemplary impression on Freud. Nevertheless, he allowed Anna's analysis to persuade him that a girl shifts her love object and rejects her mother in order to turn to her father. According to Freud, girls do not only have to change their first object, they also have to shift their pleasure zone from clitoris to vagina in order to become fully female.[20]

For Freud, Anna represented the strongest possible example of women who drastically shift objects – something that in my opinion 'normal' women do not do. She represents a deviant course of development, namely that of rejecting femininity and attempting to completely dis-identify from her mother and, instead, identify with men and become her father's squire. This object shift, having been pushed too far, is in no way the common process that Freud refers to when speaking of the female Oedipus complex. It does not lead to desiring a man but, rather, to wanting to *be* one. It is far more plausible that it concerns a homosexual or lesbian development.

According to Freud, sexual inhibition is part of the normal female Oedipus complex. The path towards femininity, as described by Freud, is so protracted that it is hard to understand how a girl ever grows into a heterosexual woman. It is no wonder, then, that Freud had difficulty answering the question: 'What does woman want?' His oedipal theory required more object shifting than he was able to conclude – apart from Anna – as he did, indeed, realize and admit in 1931. He acknowledges that his ideas concerning this object shift are based on 'women who have a very strong attachment to the father'.

Freud seems relieved that he would not, after all, need to revise his theory about the Oedipus complex as the core of neurosis. The 'normality' of women who shift objects is not convincing to me. Yet, Freud thought that women who do not shift objects are neurotic. This may well be based on a different and irritating personal experience: on the tough resistance he encountered in disengaging Martha, his wife, from her mother.

In the end, Freud came to the conclusion that in women the negative Oedipus complex – the love for the parent of the same sex – forms the core of the neurosis. The germ of subsequent paranoia in the woman lies in the pre-oedipal relationship with the mother. Indeed, the fear of being murdered or 'greedily eaten' by the omnipotent mother is far from rare.[21]

Attachment to the mother

Instead of shifting objects, the girl frequently remains attached to the first object, albeit with mixed feelings. The ambivalence that began in her earliest childhood intensifies during adolescence, is tangible in the adult woman, and can rage on into old age. It is possible, too, that she may transfer her ambivalent relationship with her mother to her daughter, as was the case with Nora. Separation does not play the same role for the girl as it does for the boy, nor is it for her a required condition for developing a healthy sexuality, as it is for him. Separation often comes into being only partially, without it necessarily having any negative effects on the girl's development. When separation either does not occur at all or else is radical, the result will be pathological. What I have called the 'symbiotic illusion' with regard to the mother, the hope and yearning to be one with her, is just as destructive as its opposite, as demonstrated by Electra's rage.

The happy medium between clinging and rejecting offers the best chances for a gratifying life. It seems that a certain amount of ambivalence is inevitable, with the result that girls have a hard time expressing angry feelings towards the mother – for, in spite of everything, they will always need her. They will be more inclined to silent angry outbursts and secret murderous fantasies. Girls tend to fiercely repress their aggression and direct it towards themselves rather than towards the other – hence female masochism.[22]

The combination of love and hatred for the same parent, as is the case for the girl, is, as I mentioned earlier, far more fateful than what occurs in the boy who desires one parent and thus sees the other as a rival. The girl will often feel threatened by her inner maternal image because she fears the revenge of her mother. She can hear her mother say that she is not nice or that she is hurt by her. That inner voice pursues her and, even as adults, many women are still afraid of their (internalized) mother – or, rather, her judgment. In my experience, masochism in women is thus more frequently related to the mother they carry within them, including all ensuing conflicts, than to the father.

Struggles around female development

According to the classical psychoanalytic theory developed by Sigmund Freud at the beginning of the twentieth century, two conditions were to be met before femininity could be attained. First of all, the girl had to shift 'erogenous zones': the place of physical desire had to move from the clitoris to the vagina. Second, she needed to shift the object of her love from mother to father. Thus she was required to relinquish two essential sources of gratification in order to become a woman. Actually, she had to relinquish her original masculinity, her clitoral masturbation in the phallic phase, to be able to attain true femininity.

In Freud's opinion the girl was a little man before becoming a woman. He was supported in this concept by his young Dutch colleague Jeanne Lampl-de Groot.[23] In 1927, she published an article – for which Freud provided a highly laudatory foreword – in which she reports on the girl's phallic phase. It is her position that during this phase in her development the girl loves her mother like a little boy and aspires to be her mother's husband. Sometimes this is, indeed, the case.

I remember a girl of about 5 who lived alone with her mother. Her father, with whom the mother had had a short-lived relationship and who did not live with her, had died before Barbara was born. The mother was a vain woman, entirely focused on herself, who did not tolerate another adult in her proximity. She took the child to bed with her, leaned on her, and considered her more or less an extension of her own persona, not a separate individual. Barbara came to me for therapy because she constantly wanted to see her father's photograph and wanted her mother to read her the fairytale of Sleeping Beauty every day, as if the father had to be reawakened so as to intervene. The child was completely affixed to her mother, acting like her mother's lover. It was obviously a collusion that accommodated the mother's yearnings. Thus, this attitude in daughters does occur, but not as commonly as Lampl-de Groot assumed.

Since, according to Freud, the only libido was the male libido, the girl was born a small man. Just like the boy, she went through a phallic phase with a male sex organ that, unfortunately, turned out to be much too small – namely, the clitoris. In order to become feminine, she had to go through a psychic castration, comparable to the physical counterpart, the clitoridectomy, which is still performed in some cultures. She had to abandon any form of gratification and go through a metamorphosis.

On his way to masculinity, such sacrifices were not expected of the boy, since he was born fully as a man. 'The constitution [of the woman] will not adapt to its function without any resistance', Freud wrote.[24] In his eyes, the girl was, on the one hand, more bisexual and, on the other, less feminine and not quite as natural as the boy: 'Nature takes her claims into less careful account than is the case with masculinity.' The boy need not shift love objects, need not shift his sexual feelings, nor alter his masculine attitude. Recent research has amply demonstrated once again that this opinion is largely culturally determined. In Freud's time it was already abundantly clear that there were not enough nerve bundles in the vagina to make the totally unnecessary switch from clitoris to vagina.[25] The fact that he clung to this, nevertheless, had to do with a centuries-old prejudice against the female genitalia as a derivative of the male.

In the 1920s, a vehement discussion concerning female development began among psychoanalysts.[26] Among other things, the question arose whether both sexes did not actually begin life by being feminine rather than masculine. After all, early in life the boy also identifies with the mother. A number of researchers assumed that there is an authentic – even a primary – femininity in both boys and girls.[27] In the meantime, this issue has been settled in favour of pioneers who were opposed to Freud. Therefore it is not the girl who starts life as a boy, but the boy who has to find his sexual identity by dis-identifying with his mother.

Freud believed that the girl does not become a woman until puberty, when she discovers her vagina and completely abandons the 'male' clitoris. Today, psychoanalysts agree that, from earliest childhood on, both sexes not only develop a male or female sexual identity and its accompanying role pattern, but they are also bound to have at least an intuitive knowledge of the vagina, and that the denial of the existence of the vagina, by small boys as well as some adult men, is thus a sign of fear and resistance.[28] The corresponding desire to penetrate or be penetrated, respectively, exists in the preconscious of the boy and the girl. It is now generally accepted that she is already conscious of erotic feelings quite early on, both in her internal and external genitalia, particularly in her vagina and clitoris. It is self-evident that little children do not spend much time worrying about the concept of gender – they simply want to have everything, be everything, and be able to do everything, a concept of omnipotence that has to be abandoned at the cost of a great deal of narcissistic anguish.

When at around the age of 1 or 2 children discover the difference between the sexes, this is not just a milestone in their development, but a blow to their sense of self-worth as well, a narcissistic affront to which both sexes react with a passing phase of penis envy or fear of injury.[29] These days, when such reactions continue or are too intense, this is seen as a reaction to previous – pre-genital, namely oral or anal – frustrations that the girl, in particular, experiences with regard to her mother or caregiver. A phallic phase in which the girl behaves like a little boy was not confirmed in an extensive study,[30] nor was the negative oedipal phase in which Jeanne Lampl-de Groot believed, with Freud's warmest approval.[31]

Today the longing to have a child is no longer seen as a substitute for penis envy but as an authentic female longing. Far more finely tuned thought is devoted to penis envy these days. It is no longer merely a metaphor, but also an encapsulating term for a series of problems having to do with narcissism and self-appreciation. In the adult woman it is not a rock-solid unalterable given that cannot be analysed, as Freud formulated it, but a symptom, a sign that points to problems, such as denying the vagina, and this qualifies for treatment.[32]

Following Freud and theoretically worked out by the French psychoanalyst Jacques Lacan, French psychoanalysis uses the phallus as signifier (*significant*) of what they call the 'symbolic order'. It is a developmental stage that applies to both sexes, whereby, so it is thought, phallic monism – the belief that there is only one sex – continues to play a role in both genders. The term 'phallus' is here not used to refer to a body part but is intended as a symbol. This symbol refers to the attainment of a developmental phase in which it becomes clear that not every desire can be fulfilled. The two genders look like two halves that, according to Plato, were one and must now find each other because each one alone is incomplete.

Freud rightfully called attention to the problem of bisexuality, especially in girls.[33] It appears that bisexuality is less repressed in girls than in boys who, in order to become men, must suppress their identification with and love for their mothers. Thus, in contrast to what Freud believed, boys actually relinquish more than do girls. In my view, the girl's bisexuality results not so much from the fact that she must give up her so-called male organ, the clitoris, but, rather, from her persistent homosexual yearning for her first object – a yearning that a male partner cannot always, or not completely, satisfy.

Insofar as I can tell, the important question whether girls shift objects has to be answered negatively. If Sophocles and other authors were right with regard to Electra, women are often far more preoccupied with the love–hate relationship with their mother than with the oedipal love for their father. The frequently absent father is seen more from a distance and both desired and idealized, as in the case of Electra and in girls of our day. In contrast, the mother image, whether loved or hated, is ever-present, both in reality and in the girl's mind's eye. The mother is blamed for not being a satisfying love object for the girl[34] and, furthermore, for getting in the way of the girl's relationship with her father. This leads to a split between the frustrating 'bad' mother, on the one hand, and the idealized 'good' father figure, on the other. Thus, as metaphor, Electra seems to me to be more suitable than Oedipus to the problematic aspects of female development.

Mother and daughter caught between attraction and aversion

Like Oedipus, Electra is an extreme, a perversion of the average fantasy. A girl can move between two poles, each equally destructive and pathological, without shifting objects. She can reject her first object and turn away from her mother defensively, filled with hatred and aversion, in order to escape from the fear of being devoured, as was the case with Electra.

To give, first, an example of aversion: Eva, a well-educated young woman, came to me and wanted me to speak with her mother. Meanwhile, she herself had broken off all contact with her mother. Through my questions she began to realize that she had not freed herself from her mother in the least, as she thought she had, and that she would do better to find the solution to her problems in herself rather than in her mother. She then wept for a week, felt better, and decided she wanted to start treatment. After a few conversations, Eva told me that she used to wake up every night in a cold sweat, but that suddenly this was no longer happening. Apparently, the fear of her mother had decreased since we had discussed it. A manifest avoidance, as with Eva, usually goes hand in hand with a latent obsession with everything that is linked to the mother and to motherhood.

The other equally extreme outcome of the daughter dilemma is that the daughter remains stuck in a closely knit symbiotic attachment to the mother. Usually this is repeated from generation to generation and occurs in mothers who have not resolved their own attachment to their own mothers and subsequently use their daughters as narcissistic extensions of themselves. This often ends up as a combination of love and hate, so that the anger with the mother is projected onto the daughter, with all the concomitant guilt feelings. The mother–daughter mirroring may engender the feeling that they are responsible for one another's well-being and, consequently, for one another's destruction.

These two extremes – namely, turning away from the mother and continuing to be intimately linked with her, or an alternating version thereof – only appear to be different. That which looks different at the level of behaviour can amount to the same thing on the inner (intra-psychic) level. However, neither extreme includes an object shift from mother to father.

Fathers and daughters

Being focused on the mother does not alter the fact that the father exerts a strongly erotic attractive force on the girl, and that she starts flirting with men at quite an early age.[35] Girls exhibit libidinous feelings for their fathers from their first year on, far earlier than classical psychoanalytic theory had assumed.[36] Because of conflicts with the mother, the father is sought out as an alternative and idealized, which may resemble an object shift. As mentioned before, in that sense a split often occurs that makes the father the good parent and the mother the bad one. Fathers have to make up for what has gone wrong with mothers.

Another important function of the father is that, for both boys and girls, he can serve as an identification object that acknowledges the child's need for independence and sexual identity. Generally, men are more aware of their own desires than are women. A father is more inclined to mould the world to his will and takes the initiative more readily than mothers do.[37]

Boys can see their fathers as rivals. This is different for girls: the aggression that originates in the relationship with the mother has to be suppressed. When she tries to woo the father, she cannot direct her hostility towards him. With the love and hate that is hers, she is fearful of hurting him. The sadism that remains from the oral and anal struggle with her mother may inadvertently find its way to him. Consequently, she is afraid of forfeiting both his and her mother's love. Once again, her guilt feelings will drive her to curb her aggressive impulses.[38]

The father's function as the one who recognizes the girls' femininity acquires a new impulse during her adolescence. On the one hand, he must appreciate the girl as a woman, on the other, he must not conduct himself as a seducer, and the line between these is exceedingly thin. The girl needs his attention and words of praise in order to feel appreciated as a woman. In that respect, Agamemnon failed in his duty, just as many fathers do today. The father may compensate for, or correct, the relationship with the mother. He is providing a second chance, but that could also end in a double disappointment, with detrimental results for the girl, for her sense of self-worth, and for her ability to enter into stable heterosexual object relationships.

On the whole, a girl is less absolute and more forgiving in the demands she makes on her father than she is with her mother, because she has a far more archaic bond with the latter, as Electra demonstrates. She idealizes her father in the hope of finally actualizing the idyll that was missing with her mother. During adolescence, a daughter will be inclined to free herself from the father far more successfully than she ever did with regard to the mother. The suggestion of an erotic connection can be frightening, both for her and for him.

From daughter to woman

The woman recreates herself in her own image, and the results of that situation can be clearly retraced in her development. The heavily charged combination of love and hate for one and the same parent and the idealization of the other is nowhere better reflected than in the Electra myth. The mother–daughter relationship is central here, in contrast to the Oedipus myth, on which Freud – who discovered the Oedipus complex – bases the development of the male.

Emotional problems, such as masochism, vaginismus, frigidity, fear of fusing, and postnatal depression are closely related to the mother image that a woman has. The transmission across generations of both pathology and mental health runs with fewer disturbances in the female line, which can be an advantage as well as a disadvantage.[39]

Women begin life in a homosexual bond with the mother, their first object, with whom they share sex and gender as well as gender identity and with whom they will identify throughout many subsequent phases of life. 'Identification need not hamper separation. Healthy feminine development would call for both a positive identification with the mother as woman along with an emotional separation from her in the interest of individuation and establishing one's own identity as woman–wife–mother' (Meissner, p. 38).[40] In order to be able to separate, girls must be able to differentiate between aggression and independence, for they are going to differ from a person whom they will continue to need. With regard to their mother image, women often have to sail skilfully between the Charybdis of hate and the Scylla of symbiotic illusion.

Women need not separate as radically as men, since their sexual identity is not at stake, as it is for men. Therefore, the rejection of the mother and a radical object shift, as postulated in oedipal theory, are to be mentioned as less necessary – indeed, as quite uncommon and not at all healthy. The conclusion from all of the above might be that heterosexuality is merely added to a lifelong homosexual bond, in the sense that for the woman the mother continues to be the reference point.

Chapter 6

What does woman want?

The question Sigmund Freud posed at the end of his life, '*Was will das Weib?*' [What does woman want?] is even now a burning question that has not been robbed of its topicality in any way whatsoever. Just as art historians continue to scrutinize the 'Mona Lisa' in search of the *ewig Weibliche* [eternal feminine], so psychoanalysts keep digging into the history of female development, hoping to reveal her psyche. In spite of the divergent views, the participants in this debate agree that both the separation between mother and daughter and women's sexual development can generate problems. Moreover, restraint of aggression and feelings of guilt and shame are again and again linked to female development.[1]

A girl must accomplish two tasks in order to grow into a mature, independent, and emotionally stable woman. In the first place, she must free herself in part from the internal image of her mother, which she carries with her, both consciously and unconsciously. In addition, she has to discover her sexual feelings and accept her sexual identity so as to derive both pleasure and satisfaction from each of them.[2]

According to classical psychoanalytic theory, a woman was not born but made. A successful development of her femininity depended on four basic changes. She had to shift erogenous zones (from clitoris to vagina), object (from mother to father), sexual identity (from little boy to little girl), and from an active to a passive position. This means that the girl would have to renounce all her original vital sources of gratification and direct herself to other, new sources so as to become a complete woman.

This improbable argument, not based on the available knowledge of the female body, went – and goes – against elementary logic. It was founded on a symmetrical development between boys and girls that Freud assumed for a long time. It implied that his Oedipus complex, invented from a male perspective, *mutatis mutandis*, had to be true for women as well. Just as the little boy desires his mother and sees his father as a rival, so the little girl longs for her father and sees the mother as rival – so stated classical theory.

Up to this point, we have been able to ascertain repeatedly how a genuine relationship between mother and daughter is part of a girl's development.

The sticking points on the road to femininity are primarily connected to the narrow correlation between the two above-mentioned aspects of her development – namely, separation and sexuality. The girl's first love relationship and attachment is, by definition, homosexual, in the sense of a same-sex relationship between mother and daughter. Furthermore, she must learn to handle her constantly renewed identification with this first and most important love object. The combination of these features renders a girl doubly linked to her mother instead of learning to stand on her own two feet, as the boy does. This state of affairs may or may not become a hindrance for her ability to sustain intimate relationships. The outcome will also depend on whether the mother needed a daughter who would serve as a duplicate and an extension of herself.

The essential question of the separation and individuation of women had been raised by sociologists and feminists and was then picked up by the lay press before psychoanalysis – having long shed insufficient light on mother and daughter – paid attention to it from the 1970s onward.[3]

There has been a great deal of speculation about women's psycho-sexual development for more than a hundred years now, in particular on the part of psychoanalysis, which was created around the early 1900s. At that point, for the first time, special attention was paid to women, although woman, hysteria, and psychiatry were more or less synonymous at the time (see Chapter 10).

In what follows I discuss separation and sexuality largely separately. In practice, they are obviously closely connected: in a positive sense when sexual development promotes separation, in a negative sense when an obstructed separation becomes a deterrent to the girl's sexual development.

From the very start, a girl tends to foster strongly contradictory yearnings. On the one hand, she would like to be independent and develop her own identity; on the other, she yearns for a reunification with her mother. If she is not capable of resolving this dilemma, she may remain in the situation I have called symbiotic illusion. Since women reproduce themselves, each deficiency can be transferred from one generation to the next. The same is true for the failure of separation.

The fact that, in my view, no object shift takes place has serious consequences for an insight into the female Oedipus complex, which deserves a name of its own – hence the term Electra complex. Neither Freud nor any of his followers paid sufficient attention to the implications of an oedipal phase that for girls does not run parallel to that of boys.

Breaking free from parents is and continues to be difficult

Liselotte, a young woman, came to see me because she has a boyfriend who is unkind to her and occasionally beats her, in fact. She suffers from misgivings around every little thing and is certainly incapable of deciding whether she should or should not break off the relationship. She 'loves her boyfriend', although she disparages him. Moreover, she adds that 'there can be no fucking' because when the boyfriend penetrates her he loses his erection – a problem he has had for twenty years.

Liselotte is equally unable to free herself from her parents, kind, well-meaning people who, according to her, always know better what decision she ought or ought not to make. They provide her with everything her heart desires. She can certainly be categorized as spoiled and that keeps her in her place as a little girl. She lives in a house that the parents purchased for the children, and there is a good deal of contact back and forth because with every crisis she falls back on home and on advice from her parents. She can never say no to her parents' wishes concerning her plans and her lifestyle.

As I was wondering what caused Liselotte to be so masochistic, I heard her say that, in her eyes, her opinion never counted for anything and that she felt she was never taken seriously. As she experiences it, she has never been more than an instrument of the good intentions of her solicitous and overprotective parents. I assume that Liselotte has unconsciously come to see herself as the victim of this configuration, to which she now seems to be giving free rein with her partner. Subsequently she tells her parents how badly he treats her, whereupon they counsel her vehemently against continuing the relationship with him. She has never properly separated from either her mother or her father.

As stated before, these parents did what they could to be there for Liselotte, the result being that she has taken a childlike position. This young woman illustrates that parents play a role in a decision such as that of leaving home by feeding the fantasies from which the child fashions her own story.

Hanna, an older woman of about 70, returned for treatment after she had spent years in analysis with someone else. Her masochistic sexual fantasies have never disappeared. It turns out that her analyst linked this fantasy primarily with the oedipal relationship with the father and the explanation provided for it by Freud. This masochism points to a homo-erotic, albeit negative, bond with the mother, which had never been discussed – all this while Hanna had a mother whom she describes as extremely strict, someone who would actually give her a thrashing when she dared to disobey. She was never able to express the hate she felt for her mother, and thus she punished herself instead.

Separation from the mother is never absolute, nor is that necessary, but it does make women more readily inclined to masochism. Anger and feelings of guilt often remain unresolved and are swallowed for fear of losing the mother's love.

It can be an unhealthy situation when no separation occurs between a girl's self-image and the image she has of her mother. This may happen when the girl never raises her voice at her mother, not even during adolescence, or does not dare to bring up a controversial topic of conversation. These kinds of girls have never contradicted their mother, not even while growing up. The silent, self-evident bond of infancy is continued without any further ado, without any interruption or rupture. They see the disruption, not to mention the break, of the implicit bond created from earliest childhood, as too terrifying. In the daughter's imagination, just a very tentative first protest would lead immediately to a breakdown in her far too vulnerable mother who, at the same time, inevitably rules over her.

Not long ago, I was travelling through India with an English family for a few days and inadvertently witnessed the conflicts that took place in utter silence. The daughter, Fenely, an intelligent, well-educated young woman who lived on her own and had travelled a great deal by herself, unwillingly went back to old patterns during the trip, which was a gift from her parents. On a practical level, the mother was efficient and caring. In addition, she was so dynamic and cheerful – never tired, always chatting about all sorts of trivia, and taking pride in her never-ending energy – that the daughter, coughing and visibly in pain due to an ear infection, did not dare to protest the pace imposed by the mother. The father, a friendly man, followed along behind them somewhat awkwardly with his pigeon toes, never offering any counter-balance. When he said anything with which his wife disagreed, he instantly withdrew his opinion and then sided with her. Not once did he defend his daughter's interests.

When I asked Fenely how she was doing, she admitted to me that she felt terribly ill but that her mother could not stand illness or weakness and so she was not going to mention it. Her vacation was totally ruined, however. The mother was an amicable, friendly woman until someone went against her wishes, at which point a deep wrinkle would form in her forehead and her mouth would turn down sourly, so I kept myself at a suitable distance.

Of course, like any child, the daughter had her own share in such an unhealthy interaction. Fenely herself provoked her mother's excessive interference with her, if only by not resisting and not showing how unpleasant certain things were for her. As the youngest, she was known as 'the baby' and, undoubtedly, took delight in this role herself.

In normal development, too, the separation between mother and daughter is more problematic than the one between mother and son. The similarity in physical and psychic sexual identity creates an insufficient difference whereby, from both sides, the relationship with the daughter offers many more points of contact for identification *without* separation. Masochism is closely linked not only to aggression but also to the taboo around sexuality. Taking pleasure in one's own body can be a source of painful fantasies when a girl has the feeling that her pleasure with a third party will be at the expense of her mother or will hurt her. Such a daughter believes that when she does not make herself entirely available to her mother, she is not a good daughter. Once this idea has taken root, it may actually cause the daughter to abandon all erotic desires.

In an unsuccessful separation, this fantasy can also exist in men and will then lead to a weak male identity. In both boys and girls it amounts to their feeling that even now their body belongs not to them, but to their mother. Therefore she has the right to manipulate them, treat them as a children, not listen to their opinion, and never let them be right. Thus it is crucial to learn to put the omnipotent mother of one's childhood into perspective – something that women find more difficult than men. Besides, the girl and the adult woman generally continue to feel much more responsible for the trials and tribulations of the mother than the boy and the man will.

It is self-evident that for the female baby the first relationship is of a narcissistic nature, for mother and daughter have the same gender and can discern their own reflection in the other. At birth every child, whether boy or girl, is confronted by a pattern of expectations and fantasies that were already created during the mother's pregnancy. These imaginings also depend on the mother's inner structure, on her family, and on the culture in which she lives. However, the pipedreams around expected babies are differently charged depending on whether they concern sons or daughters. A girl may fulfil the mother's wish to be reborn as more beautiful, better, and more perfect. A pregnant woman who is herself insufficiently separated may have the feeling that she is carrying her own mother in her womb, or else project herself so much into the foetus that she is back inside her mother's womb, as it were. If a woman lacks solid self-awareness, she might hope for a daughter as an improved version of herself.

Every woman relives her own relationship with her mother in a little daughter. The relationship with the mother is reactualized.[4] The inner theatre of the mother–daughter pair that had been created in the previous generation is played out again in the next. Various more or less healthy solutions of former conflicts are conceivable. For instance, it can be painful when the young mother frantically tries to handle motherhood differently from her own mother. She is then using her baby to straighten something out or to justify herself, and her child serves to help her to distance herself from the image she has of her mother. She wants to prove she is not just as good a mother, but actually a better one than her own, who raised her and whom she has internalized.

Another inheritance from the past is conscience. It can be more or less tolerant, strict, or judgmental and finds its origin in the internalized parents. The child appropriates their commands and taboos. But the image that we form of reality does not run parallel to reality. The inner parent is the image that was shaped during childhood and that we carry with us throughout our lives. A parent may be experienced as strict without the reality necessarily matching that image. In any event, a stern conscience is a heavy burden that is sometimes projected onto one's own child.

When the little girl becomes the embodiment of that conscience, she thus fans the fire of her mother's hatred. The child may represent the mother's angry mother and make her feel guilty when she is unable to calm her crying infant. She experiences the crying like an accusation: you're not doing it right, you're not a nice mother. On the other hand, a mother may recognize herself readily in the needy, angry baby. The child may thus become the incarnation of a daughter who will never love her mother – as a patient explained to me – because she herself never loved her own mother.

Some women make precisely those demands of themselves to which their mother was unable to respond. Some daughters have to provide the love that was lacking in their mother's life. What happens then is a reversal of the generations: the mother becomes the child that wants to be mothered by her daughter. The daughter must provide all the support and love for which her mother yearned as a child and for which she still yearns. Turning the relationships between the generations upside down, exchanging the role of mother and daughter, results in the daughter feeling guilty because she is incapable of offering her mother everything she lacks.

On the basis of this scenario, the girl, now herself a mother, may have the feeling that she is failing. It seems to her that demands are being made of her from two sides. She is being pulled both ways and cannot satisfy either her child or her mother. As a mother, she feels incompetent because she cannot give what she never received herself, but if she were able to do so, chances are that the baby would make her envious.

All these fantasies can be at play repeatedly throughout the course of a daughter's life. With regard to the separation in particular, the sometimes extremely ambivalent feelings surrounding the mother–daughter relationship are not only decisive factors but can also endure for several generations. Even in the most normal development the separation between mother and daughter seems to be more problematic than that between mother and son. The mutual similarities and the lack of gender difference provide an ample opportunity for mother and daughter to mutually identify without separation. The continued existence of a primary identification hampers the formation of a separate identity and individuality. And if there are problems around the separation, they will continue to return throughout the woman's entire development. Each new developmental phase that goes hand in hand with a step towards greater independence also gives cause for renewed identifications.

A lengthy rapprochement crisis takes place in girls – a period of approaching and withdrawing, a kind of hold-on-to-me-let-me-go period. To the toddler who takes its first steps away from the mother it is plainly noticeable that its experimentation with proximity and distance can stir fear in the mother, which is more truly the case with girls than with boys. The girl, on her part, has a double reproach to make against her mother, according to the French psychoanalyst Janine Chasseguet-Smirgel.[5] Not only has the mother deprived her of the breast, but she has also failed to provide her with a penis. The mother is omnipotent and, according to the psychoanalyst Melanie Klein, has every sex organ at her disposal, at least in the child's fantasy. The daughter's vehement envy of and sadism against her mother – which she must manage to conceal – give rise to extra guilt feelings in the girl towards her mother.

The more the little girl notices that this aspiration displeases her mother and may even frighten her, the more will she begin to feel more ambivalent and more uneasy about her need for independence. Obviously, she is afraid to lose her mother's love – all the more, or more justifiably so, when her mother seems unable to cope with her daughter's experiments in running off. It is on the basis of whether this phase passes harmoniously or discordantly that the inner mother-and-child pair, which the woman must carry with her throughout life, is created.

In the interim, research has amply affirmed that generally a girl has a more ambivalent relationship with her mother than a boy does. This happens less because she blames her mother for not having given her a penis than because of separation difficulties, whereby she can readily experience the bond with her mother as an oppressive one, especially when this connection has run its course weighted down with ambivalence and dissatisfaction. The period when the toddler is experimenting with distance from the mother also happens to be the time that toilet training takes place, which can readily turn into a power struggle both in reality and in fantasy. Frightening experiences concerning the child's own body go hand in hand with this, such as loss of control and the letting go of 'treasured' internal products. Feelings of shame and the sense of being nothing more than a waste product, dirty or even undesired, are pre-eminently linked to this phase.[6] Frustrations of oral desires, eating problems, and fights about eating or not eating, as with Nora's little daughter in Chapter 5, may cause rage and hatred. Toilet training, often a power struggle, can also turn into a source of frustration, complete with feelings of hatred and anal-sadistic preoccupations. By projecting her pent-up anger, the girl is afraid of revenge from her mother's end, a revenge that does not tally with reality but is enacted in the girl's fantasy. The external reality is always just a part of our reality. The deciding factor is the psychic or inner reality, which can have a very different appearance.

In her imagination, the girl may see a mother who threatens to harm her if she will not satisfy her wishes. She starts to fear for the vulnerable internal part of her body, and for a girl the genitalia are intricately tied up with this. If she does not obey, the mother could destroy her, poison or demolish her, as in the evil fairy tales. Apart from their innate sensitivity as babies[7] (girls react more sensitively to interactions with the mother from the very start), girls are more compliant and are toilet-trained earlier. From a social point of view (speech included), girls develop faster than boys. Apart from a biologically determined predisposition, this compliance can be the result of her early identification with the mother, on the one hand, and of her fear of losing the mother's love on the other: after all, the girl needs the mother to set herself free from her.

For various reasons, the girl tends to feel deprived or slighted. Rightfully or wrongfully, she may feel that she is unable to fulfil the mother's longings. She is not a boy, and she feels that she can only satisfy the mother by offering herself as her extension. This is one way the girl's unconscious conviction may show itself. She easily imagines that she should have been a boy, or that a brother is her mother's favourite and is given preferential treatment. This will arouse intense jealousy in her, at which point the girl is at a double disadvantage: first of all, she is not her mother's privileged love object and, second, she is not encouraged to free herself like the boy, who is – and is permitted to be – different. She need not become 'different' from the mother, she follows in her mother's footsteps and therefore may resemble her. This identification can take place with or without separation.

For the girl, the vicissitudes of separation are both important and potentially burdensome. On the one hand, separating is painful and laden with guilt feelings; on the other hand, it is shameful to be small and dependent on the mother, and injurious to one's sense of self as well.

Tira, a 14-year-old girl, was admitted to a clinic for adolescents because she had dropped out of school, was anxious, and stayed at home all day long with her mother. The mother, for her part, does not stimulate the separation. Although she finds the clinginess troublesome, she is also fearful and overprotective. Tira wages a bitter struggle with the psychiatrists and caregivers and does everything humanly possible to avoid being forced to do anything. The only way to maintain the feeling that she exists and is heard is to exert power through her powerlessness and obstinacy. Psychoanalytic treatment, in which her anger and anxiety were revealed with great difficulty, finally brought relief. She turned out to be intelligent and returned to school, with excellent results.

In a different scenario, the daughter may be the one who must fulfil the demands of the mother's superego (be strong but yet not too independent, make sure everyone in the family is always content, sacrifice yourself) and of the ego-ideal (the woman she had wanted to be). If such is the case, she will feel doubly responsible for her mother's ups and downs – at the cost of herself, if need be.

Such a woman is Lara, who is young, married, and the mother of a little girl, and who is exhausted because she must always be cheerful. She thinks she should be available day and night to her mother and grandmother whom she pities because they spent the war years in a Japanese camp in Indonesia, something they never speak about but have never come to terms with either. Her mother always denied the misery in the world and created an unrealistic, fairytale-like atmosphere in her environment that was at odds with reality. The mother's marriage was hardly any less dreadful for her than the camp. She had married a man who abused her psychologically and physically, but she only divorced him much later, when the children had already left home. Lara always comes to her sessions with me with a broad smile on her face, as if she is always happy and cheerful. She often wonders if she is not in the way, if I am ill, tired, hungry, or otherwise unwell and need her help. She then treats me as if I am her needy, traumatized mother or grandmother.

Sigmund Freud assumed that the formation of the female conscience was inadequate. The development of an independent conscience gets stuck because the girl does not free herself from the mother and then from the father. She does not overcome her Oedipus complex as the boy does. Thus, according to Freud, her conscience does not gain the strength and independence that would confer cultural significance on it. A female Moses would be unimaginable for Freud. This is different for a man, whose conscience he refers to as 'the heir of the Oedipus complex', which he had to conquer, after all. He develops his strong conscience by renouncing the mother and identifying with the father. This point of view concerning the fragile female conscience was based on prejudice. The story is more complex. Because the girl is afraid to gamble away her mother's love, she behaves herself, she is a good girl, she obeys. She projects or swallows her anger, which makes her mother appear stricter than she really is. As a result of these projections and introjections, which are a legacy of the earlier ambivalent bond with the mother, the female superego is, on the one hand more demanding of the self: her conscience is formed very early on and is therefore more archaic than that of the man; on the other, the female conscience is more indulgent towards others, but it is certainly not weaker or of lesser moral calibre, as Freud believed.[8]

The consequences of the bond with the mother manifest themselves in another area as well. A mother who is not happy with herself, her gender, her sexuality – in short, an insecure mother – can easily generate similar feelings in her daughter. A girl is likely to attribute her mother's unfulfilled longings for love and admiration to her own shortcomings. If she thinks that she would be better able to satisfy her mother's longings if she were a boy, this may be a reason for her to adopt a male attitude.

Some daughters cling to their mother in anger or despair and remain tied to her in a lifelong love–hate relationship. Contradictory desires to fuse and disassociate keep alternating. The result may also be that any form of dependency is rejected, or vice versa – as in the symbiotic illusion – that becoming even a little detached does not succeed at all.

The course of the separation process is of crucial importance and can be pathogenic for both mother and daughter. It bears repeating: often the girl already experiences any inclination to separation or autonomy as disloyal and aggressive towards the mother, even though she does not attack her mother in thought, let alone in word or deed. Any of this may happen because the girl assumes – often rightly – that the mother will see her daughter's process towards freedom as a threat or that it will upset her profoundly, which does often happen. All of the above can make it more difficult for a woman to marshal the positive aggression that is needed to realize her own objectives.

Lastly, there is the example of Sarah, a young Jewish woman who came for treatment because she is suffering from feelings of depression and depersonalization. She is the daughter of a woman who had lost her own mother and grandmother during the war. At the age of 14, Sarah's mother was suddenly and dramatically left by herself in Amsterdam, totally alone, in great danger, and without a place to hide. Her mother's mother had chosen to 'abandon' or 'save' her daughter – depending on one's viewpoint – in order to accompany her own mother, Sarah's great-grandmother, to a concentration camp. The great-grandmother seems to have been an extremely tyrannical widow who lived with her daughter and granddaughter. Sarah's grandmother felt she could not leave her mother and was, as a result, forced to leave her daughter behind.

When Sarah's mother herself had a child, she became depressed. The birth of a child, and a daughter at that, confronted her with her past all over again, with the fact that she had been abandoned and no longer had a mother to support her. On the one hand, as a daughter she was not as self-denying as her mother had been for her grandmother. Of course, anger towards her murdered mother who was no longer present to help her was equally taboo. The story of this young woman illustrates how experiences are transmitted from mother to daughter for generation after generation.

Problems having to do with separation and symbiosis reappear in a woman's life with some regularity. Each new phase in the girl's development presents new starting points.

Up to this point separation and sexuality could be discussed independently of one another, but these themes are more and more intricately intertwined as development progresses, as we shall see.

Budding sexuality

The conflicts of the girl with her mother of the first few years may continue to play tricks on her throughout her life. Sometimes they are so fierce that they lead to – mostly unconscious because guilt-laden – destructive fantasies about destruction or being destroyed. Subsequently, this can result in all kinds of physical symptoms, varying from frigidity and vaginismus to constipation and abdominal pain. Penetration is frightening, not only because of the intrusion of a foreign body but also because of the above-mentioned fantasies. In such a case, the woman is afraid of damaging the man's penis, or else, through projection, the latter turns into a dangerous and threatening object. It is remarkable how many girls in the latency period (elementary school age) – and adult women as well – have vague abdominal complaints. Such complaints frequently have to do with 'archaic fantasies' such as castration fears and fears of injury when the girl dreads the presence of a malevolent mother inside her body. The mother – who has incorporated the father's penis – will now damage the inside of her body.[9] The unconsciously perceived similarity between mouth, anus, and vagina as receptive, enveloping, contracting, or even aggressively biting organs can unleash frightening fantasies. As a result of the projection of her own anger, the little girl experiences her mother as aggressive and her own internal, hollow organs as dangerous or endangered. Furthermore, women often unconsciously link sexuality and anal phase fantasies, anal sadism in particular. After all, both anus and vagina are hollow organs that can either withhold something or let something out. Pinching off or holding back stool out of resistance to the mother can be an expression of anger and a tool in the struggle with her. This struggle is connected with unconscious anal sadistic fantasies. Every form of sadism when directed at the self provides a seed-bed for masochism.

For the girl the lack of an external, visible sex organ means the lack of an anchor that could provide her with security concerning the centre of her sexual perceptions. The boy's protruding sex organ gives him a legitimate reason to play with his penis and to touch it every time while urinating. What is permitted for boys with regard to erotics and sexuality is, as we know, often forbidden for girls, or else they interpret it as such.[10] This can cause a girl to experience both her anatomical build and the way she is being raised as a prohibition of masturbation and pleasure. Even today, girls still have less sexual freedom than boys. Besides, a girl's sexual perceptions are more diffuse and internal in nature than those of boys and are therefore harder to identify.

In addition, the existing taboos are reinforced because of the lack of a specific name for the female genital organs.[11] Generally, parents do not make a clear distinction between the various functions. The anal, urethral, and genital area is largely referred to with some vague term: parents talk about 'bottom', 'in front', 'crotch', or 'down there', without differentiating. Such silence can be the result of feeling shame around an organ that lacks any demonstrable useful function. Obviously, the girl adopts this feeling of shame non-verbally, especially when she hears labia discussed as a place of shame. Generally speaking, the mother does not dare to mention the clitoris as a delectable spot to her daughter, and neither does the father.

The silence around the girl's genitals is bound to have various causes. They may to some extent be linked to the fact that the vagina has an internal, hidden location, is invisible, and as yet has no clear function. However, the same silence also rules the clitoris, despite its visibility. Possibly the parents' hesitation to discuss this organ or the pleasant sensations it can provide arises from their embarrassment to talk about enjoyment instead of functionality. In contrast to the boy's willie, which potentially has several functions (urination, experiencing pleasure, masturbation, ejaculation), the clitoris serves only for the sensation of pleasure. The girl will internalize the parents' reserve, albeit non-verbally.

It is generally accepted that toddler masturbation functions as a development stimulant. It provides the possibility of becoming master over one's own body and of separating. It is a possibility that, sadly, a girl frequently has to do without or that causes her additional fear instead of pleasure. In this regard she is less carefree than the boy and thus feels deprived. She wants to be able to make babies, just like the powerful mother, but so does the boy. She does not yet have any concrete indications that in this matter she holds the advantage.

It is not clear whether a girl is less inclined to masturbate or has less of a sense of how to go about it. One may wonder whether she is disappointed in her own genitals or whether she feels castrated because her organ is more difficult to use and play with than a boy's. Be that as it may, she appears to be far more conscious than the little boy of the prohibitive rules concerning sexual pleasure. Since she is toilet-trained earlier than the boy and the chance of confusion regarding the anal, urethral, and genital area is greater in her, the prohibitive rules can very easily extend to the entire area.

While parents tend to find masturbation in boys more or less normal, they are not quite sure how to handle it in girls. It is rare that parents spontaneously mention self-gratification in girls, unless a problem has cropped up. Compulsive playing with their willie is unusual, both in boys and in girls, although it does bring parents to seek counselling. It may be an expression of a fearful question such as 'Am I broken?' Concerned mothers do visit paediatricians to complain about their daughter's irritated vulva, or more explicitly about overt and frequent masturbation. Usually, this can be seen as a concern about their own genitals – both the daughter's and the mother's – and a request for further explanation, information, and reassurance. At its core are anxious, primarily unconscious questions and fantasies around sexuality. The phenomenon probably has little to do with the attainment of genital pleasure as such: rather, it indicates the young girl's desperate search for what is missing (visible genitals) and the mother's inability to handle this. It is self-evident that the mother's experience with her femininity has an enormous influence on the daughter. Insecurity and a poor sense of self-worth are readily transmitted from mother to daughter.

In the latency period, the fantasies around body and sexuality normally decrease in intensity because school and learning fully occupy the girl's attention. For girls it is sometimes a matter of a taboo of knowledge or inhibition concerning the exploration of the world. Boys have greater freedom here and often do more exploring. As toddlers they play more freely with their genitals, explore them extensively, and chat about them. The inhibition of girls may be linked to a supposed prohibition to touch the genitals or to mention them by name. The fact that the girl's genitals are for the most part hidden should also play a role in her development. I return to the denial of the female genitalia and the connection with vagueness in thinking about them in the chapter on hysteria (Chapter 10). Learning can be difficult because of restrained curiosity, and mathematics is more often a problem for girls than for boys. Symbolically, splitting may refer to aggression (fractions and fracturing), while a lack in spatial understanding may refer to confusion about the image that the child has formed of its own body (also known as 'body schema'). Generally speaking, exploration of the outside world can lag behind more internally directed female interest.[12] Girls are more inclined towards introspection than boys because they are more inner- than outer-directed, both literally and figuratively.

In the latency period, 'female docility' usually has the upper hand. Astrid Lindgren, for example, saw this very clearly and thus created a naughty little girl – Pippi Longstocking – who turns the good little girl image upside down. The proverbial docility of little girls, usually a source of delight for parents as well as teachers and generally applauded by society, has to do with the extreme adaptation of the girl to the demands of the (inner) mother. Often she is a model of neatness, cleanliness, modesty, and lack of aggressiveness. Playing with her own genitals does not quite fit into this self-image, especially because in masturbation the fantasy is more important than the act. It is an outlet for all kinds of feelings and frustrations. Sadomasochistic masturbation fantasies are the reason why girls often renounce self-gratification out of a sense of guilt towards the mother or out of shame.[13]

The relative equilibrium of the latency period will be disrupted by the subsequent more turbulent phase, at least in a positive development. At the start of pre-puberty – at around the age of 8 to 10, depending on internal and external circumstances – docility begins to make space for a more ambivalent attitude towards the mother. At the same time, the girl's attachment to the mother and her dependency on her – in short, her symbiotic longings – are intensified.

The girl wonders: do I prefer being a boy among the boys or a girl among the girls? She feels attracted to girls, but to boys as well. The desire to be both boy and girl presents itself again, while the impossibility thereof begins to dawn. In short, bisexual fantasies increase, and that can result in insecurity around one's own body. A safe and familiar homosexual focus on the mother is reinforced by challenges that are both exciting and threatening to the equilibrium. Libidinous enticements directed at the father and heterosexuality create the need to break away from the mother. The girl is confused, she has intense mood swings, and crying jags are not at all unusual. She reacts to all of this by falling back into old and more familiar behavioural patterns such as hiding behind her mother. Attachment alternates with its opposite, anger and outbursts of rage. It is a contradiction and a disequilibrium that many mothers do not know how to handle.

In this prelude to adolescence, sexuality begins to play a role again in the background, and once more the mother's example becomes important. Sexuality readily falls under the prohibition of 'impurity' – confusion with anal eroticism is not unusual – and gives rise to feelings of shame and guilt. The girl tries to prevent rejection, for she is deathly afraid of losing her mother as support and identification object in this new phase. Internally she is flung between tender love for her mother and fierce feelings of hatred. It is harder for her to accept the renewed taboo of 'impurity', now known as sexuality.

She tends to deny feelings of guilt and shame that may emerge towards her mother. Her instability is expressed in altercations about seemingly trivial issues and conflicts around discipline and neatness, such as cleaning her room.

The physical changes that occur in the girl's body during puberty – developing breasts, the onset of menstruation – can cause her to feel frightened and ashamed instead of proud. These changes make her more of a rival of her mother long before she is able to enter emotionally into relationships with men: she has the looks of a mature woman, but internally she is still a small, timid girl. Although the oedipal struggle and rivalry with the mother are gaining new life, the girl simultaneously feels the need to hide behind her like a child because of all the demands that she cannot yet satisfy emotionally.

With the onset of menstruation, confusion around the female genitals increases. A revival of childlike sexual theories and anal preoccupations – particularly the cloaca theory, in which there is only one organ, one single opening, where all (sexual and excretion) functions take place – may result in a girl's rejection of her body as unattractive and dirty, and seeing herself as despicable and undesirable. The former feelings of shame come back to life again. In my practice I quite frequently encounter well-groomed grown women who tell me they are afraid that they are dirty or smell bad.

There is no inherent reason why menstruation, and its accompanying use and choice of tampons and sanitary napkins, as well as physical hygiene or the knowledge of sexual functions could not be a source of understanding and emancipation.[14] Nor is there any reason why the mother could not be of support during this process. However, for such a 'positive' development it must be assumed that the body and all bodily functions and perceptions can be freely thought about and discussed. If the body is weighed down by taboos and archaic fantasies, the danger exists that it will produce aversion instead of becoming a source of satisfaction. The development of a healthy narcissism and self-confidence and pride in being a woman is not self-evident.

The girl's sexuality is heavily influenced by the health of the mother–daughter relationship or the seriousness of the problems with her mother in early childhood. This means that the longing for a man and the possible desire to give birth to a child – that is to say, in oedipal terms, the longing for the father, the desire to receive a penis inside herself, the fantasy of giving him a child – can also be dreaded. The girl can sense any or all of this as aggression instead of a loving exchange. The father may be seen as aggressive. Other than the fact that some fathers may actually give cause for the above, it may also happen that the fears around a mother, who may be felt to be intrusive, subsequently end up being projected onto the father. Similarly, anger against the mother can easily be shifted over to the father. Hostile feelings towards the mother had to be controlled previously, which is no less true for comparable feelings towards the father later on. This causes the girl to confront double guilt feelings and an increased inhibition of aggression, directed both at the mother and the father.

If the fear of putting the mother off her stride or of destroying her is already present, then that same emotional disposition can lead to fear of damaging the father, of treating him badly. Unconscious fantasies such as seizing the father's penis, devouring it, or damaging it in some other way is a taboo that can lead to sexual inhibitions. The curtailment of hostility readily causes a projection of one's own aggression onto the other. Such a solution renders the other person dangerous – the father, or men in general.

The danger that sexual development incites is traditionally felt much more strongly in girls, by both parents and children. The budding girl often arouses erotic feelings in her father, from which both parties tend to flee. The mother may feel threatened in her womanhood by this new rival, which may go so far as to make her jealous of her daughter. Some mothers try to stay young, to participate and become the girlfriend of their daughter, as if they themselves were adolescents again. Other mothers try to attract the attention of the daughter's boyfriends.

Furthermore, fear of sexuality is also still very closely linked to fear of an unwanted pregnancy. Consciously or not, this preoccupies both mother and daughter. Under favourable conditions, mother and daughter will not avoid the body in their conversations together. On the contrary, they may well discuss menstruation, sexuality, the pill, and all else around the female body about which the girl may have questions and mother and daughter can have a chat, although many mothers still find this extremely unusual and uncomfortable.

The psychic equilibrium is once again rattled when physical development advances and a new impulse forward in the form of sex hormones makes itself known inwardly. During adolescence – the period between puberty or sexual maturity and adulthood – the girl will be better able to go her own way and free herself from old bonds. Rivalry with the mother may hamper this. Unresolved conflicts in the mother–daughter relationship often result in the girl's attempt to create distance. She simultaneously longs for fusion with her mother and fears it as a threat to her freedom. Alicia, an adolescent who has been living with her mother since the parents divorced, does nothing but pick arguments with her. She does not do her homework, she gets one failing mark after another, hangs out in coffee shops after school, and rants and raves at her mother about the slightest matters. She objects to everything and is impossible to live with, which is how she tries to demonstrate her freedom and independence. A threatening pull backwards, back to the child she was, is what she tries to resist at any cost. A pretend separation is lurking.

Gradually it becomes clear to the girl that the sexual organs have a dual function and serve for both procreation and sexual pleasure. Once the girl is sexually mature, the clitoris still serves no purpose other than pleasure. The

vagina has grown more sensitive during puberty and can better fulfil a pleasure function. Because this organ also plays an essential role in procreation, it
acquires a two-fold function, while it is equally connected to menstruation.
These various functions can easily create confusion. In addition to eroticism,
the vagina plays the role of entrance and exit in procreation. These two
functions have to be considered separately, while in the girl's fantasy a certain
connectedness needs to be maintained as well.

I once noticed on a hospital maternity ward that sexual organs were being
very freely discussed. I had never heard them talked about quite so openly by
any women before: the openness was apparently connected to the completely
non-erotic functions these body parts suddenly fulfilled. They had been
deprived of their heavily laden eroticism and thus become nameable.

The most important obstacle the young woman needs to overcome is perhaps the threatening repression of the clitoris and of gratification in general.
Both in everyday life and in classical psychoanalysis there are prejudices
against an organ that provides carefree pleasure without being in the least
useful. This pleasure often has to be ignored and even denied. In almost every
culture, female desires trigger unconscious fears of woman's insatiability. The
myth of the bacchanalian licentious horde infers the threatening effect that it
unconsciously seems to express for men. Women's fear of their own genitals
is reinforced by men's fear about them. This varies, from fear of being swallowed up or of vanishing inside a huge hole to fear of biting vaginas, of
castration, and of physical harm in general, which is associated, among other
things, with menstrual blood. All of this readily leads to a general taboo on
femininity, which exists to varying extents in many cultures.

During adolescence, the girl may develop her sense of self-worth, feel beautiful and attractive, spruce herself up, and go out to see the effect she has on
men. It is an experimental phase in which both attracting and repelling is
not unusual because everything is still very new and daunting. The girl feels
like the sorcerer's apprentice in the tale by the eighteenth-century German
writer Johann Wolfgang von Goethe, who cannot remember how to stop the
violence of the wildly flowing water once it has been unleashed.

Confused, the girl would like to escape perhaps and go back to her familiar
old home base, but the peril of the undesired fusion with the mother keeps
her from doing so. If need be, the yearning for the mother will be changed
into its opposite and expressed in hysterical aversion as the only possibility
for separation. For some girls this is the only way to protect themselves from
a terrifying fusion with the mother. However, such an almost primitive hatred
is different from the healthy aggression that is needed for separation and feeds
destructive fantasies in which every attack returns like a boomerang and
instigates fear of destruction of the personal ego.

Separation needs a healthy dose of aggressiveness. Primitive hatred feeds
the fantasy that whoever attacks one's own image will not make it out alive
oneself. If you stand up against your mother, your hand will grow from your

grave as punishment, and that evil little hand that is not allowed to masturbate does not deserve any better, so that eternal shame will be yours.

When, during this second separation–individuation phase known as adolescence, a girl is having a hard time, her guilt feelings are often mixed with archaic fears of destruction, which results in her feeling cramped and thus unable to develop her independence. Normally, a daughter will remain emotionally attached to her mother throughout adolescence, although she is protesting and freeing herself at the same time. The absence of an incest taboo, such as exists between mother and son, means, among other things, that there is no need to put a stop to physical closeness – if that has existed – and to cuddling, for example. This hold-onto-me-let-me-go attitude of girls is often hard to put up with for mothers.

The uninterrupted emotional bond of girls with their mother can have both positive and negative results. A mutually loving relationship without too much ambivalence can develop warmth and cordiality in the daughter. However, a parasitic relationship can make the daughter vulnerable, and there is a strong chance that she will transmit this problem to the next generation. She will then, in turn, develop the need for a symbiotic relationship with her children. The chance that such an unhealthy bond is generated and thereupon transmitted is greater in women than in men – women are, after all, bound to go through the same stages and phases of life as their mother did before them. This is why, even after adolescence, a daughter continues to be emotionally involved with her mother.

It is not unusual for girls to think that they are ugly – all the more so when they also have 'ugly' (in the sense of 'bad') thoughts. Their admiration of the mother will then overshadow their feeling of self-worth. My mother is beautiful and good, and I am not. Such girls tend to have the feeling that their sense of self-worth depends on the other, and they are unable to find a source of confidence inside themselves. Mothers who have difficulties, albeit unconscious, with their sexual feelings will silently transmit this message.

Obviously, there is a social and cultural aspect attached to the silence and shame surrounding sexual functions as well. Even physicians play a role in the transmission of cultural prejudices and taboos, as we can see in the fierce battle against masturbation and in the demeaning attitude towards women that is still very common in the nineteenth century and also present in Sigmund Freud's writing.[15]

Pregnancy as the culmination of female development produces renewed fantasies and preoccupations focused on the internal body. One may recall the primitive fears that surround a premature birth that can often lead to concealing the child or even killing it (as happens in many underdeveloped countries). The pregnant woman is confronted once again with the risks that falling back into old patterns brings with it[16] – she is, after all, following in her mother's footsteps. Longing or fear of fusion reappears. The daughter needs support and seeks advice from her mother or does precisely the opposite by avoiding this. The issue of separation is not simply resolved and does not disappear with adolescence.

The fear of injury that, as we have seen, was generated in the girl as a result of projecting anger can emerge again in fears around delivery and the health of the child. Is it woman's predestination that she should give birth in pain to punish her unconsciously for her passion and her creative power? It is not uncommon that this fantasy causes childbirth to be seen as a violent event of which women are afraid, for it does always hold a very real danger, as it occurs on the borderline between life and death or between living and not living.

Fears around having a child that is not right have a great deal to do with unresolved problems of aggression and guilt feelings about them, which arise from such feelings towards their own mother. At the time that she is becoming a mother, the young woman falls back on her own mother, and she feels partly like a baby again because of this. From quite a young age she senses that 'Do not do unto others what you will not have them do unto you', especially with regard to her likeness. She does not wish to resist her mother, particularly at this point in time, for if she should hurt her mother, then her own child may do the same to her, especially if it is a daughter. The act of hurting her mother might be repeated upon herself by her child. It is remarkable how many young women who have problems with their mother hope that they will not have any daughters.

Not only does the life story of her mother echo in the expectations of a girl with regard to a possible daughter, but also those of her grandmother and great-grandmother. This is all the more the case when unhealthy or failed separations have occurred in the preceding period of her life. Not only does she resemble her mother, but she may also need her again – or, vice versa, she may fear that her mother will devour her and the child, or take away the child from her because she is a competitor who is equally, or even better, able to handle things. These fears may cause her to develop a kind of 'mother phobia'.

In short, during pregnancy all the problems having to do with separation that appeared previously are coming to life again. However, if such problems were not present, or not to any serious extent, then the mother will be seen as a source of support and assistance, not as a threat.

Adèle, an introspective university-educated young woman, does not dare to ask her mother for support because the latter would take over her life completely. Yet she cannot work it out by herself either. She goes into psychotherapy because of her paralysing fear and insecurity. She has a man friend, a job, and a 2-year-old daughter, but she is habitually under severe strain. She dare not tell her parents that she has gone into analysis since that would alarm them too much. The culture at home always expected family members to solve their own problems, even though the father was being treated by a psychiatrist because of his phobias, but that had never been revealed.

Already during the first few sessions it becomes clear that Adèle's problems run across four generations of women. Her grandmother is still alive and rules the entire family. Her mother is terrified of her. Now that she has a child of her own, Adèle has grown particularly concerned. She is afraid – and rightfully so – that she will transmit the same pressure to her daughter that her mother and grandmother put on her. Nobody ever contradicts the extremely coercive grandmother. I suspect that no one is supposed to know about Adèle's treatment because the grandmother would disapprove. Everyone in the family is scared stiff of the anger of the grandmother, although Adèle's mother visits her almost every day.

In a healthy development the woman can fall back on her mother. The mother's place in her daughter's life is linked not only to the individual circumstances, but to the social ones as well, depending on milieu and ethnicity. Leaning on the mother, even telephoning her or seeing her every day, can also be seen as support instead of as a threat to independence. Nor does it need always to constitute an impediment to the establishment of the daughter's own family life.

In tracing the sexual development of girls, it becomes clear that every step forward might lead to a step backward. A girl senses that she is being pulled in opposite directions. Or, to put it differently, a girl tends to react to each progression with a regression. The separation that has already been achieved threatens to become undone. With every step in the direction of greater independence, the girl wants her mother's approval. If she does not actually see her mother, she still hears her voice. Mother's power inside her head is present even when she herself is not. That can be pleasant or menacing, depending on the relationship. Fleeing back to the mother or else avoiding her fearfully are two extremes that a girl should try hard to avoid if she does not want to lose control over her own body, her identity, and her sexuality.

As we have seen, girls' continuous repetition of their identification with their mother means that with every step forward they progressively start to resemble their mother more and more. They are going through the same phases and experiences of being-woman as their mother went through, including the menopause; thus they identify with her again and again at every step of the way. This 'separation-identification paradox'[17] is therefore an ever-recurring phenomenon and developing a personal identity is constantly threatened. Consequently, one of the most common complaints of women is their fear of resembling their own mother. Cordial or not, as an internal love-, hate-, and identification object the mother will stay with the daughter for as long as she lives.

Sometimes it happens that feelings of primitive hatred – arising in part from the repression of normal anger and guilt feelings – are repeated during treatment. This is likely to be the reason why in psychoanalysis – more than in a therapy with less frequent sessions – a primitive rage, be it overt or concealed, plays a role much more often in women than in men. The patient fears that her 'malevolent mother' will guess her intentions, will take revenge and destroy her; or, conversely, she can also have the fantasy that something dreadful will happen to her analyst (especially if she is a woman), a fantasy about which she then feels very guilty. She imagines that one of them, analyst or patient, will not make it out alive. It is my impression that such feelings are far more vehement when the woman is in treatment with a female analyst.

Women and masochism

In spite of every cultural and social change, there are fixed data that cannot be altered. It is not just biology and anatomy that set their limits. Despite all its variations, the mother–daughter relationship is an incontrovertible given as well. The survival of the primary identification, the overall following in the mother's wake, is very normal in traditional cultures and still occurs in some of Western circles as well, as exemplified by married women who have coffee with their mother every day and who prefer talking with their mother to talking with their husband. Annie asks her husband – a depressive, frightened man who is in treatment with me – to make an appointment for her, and then reluctantly comes to the phone herself. She does not arrive alone but has her husband bring her. She has no problem, she states, but her husband does, and she is here to help him. After all, *she* discusses everything with her mother. She speaks of her husband as if he were her fourth child. He is now on disability benefits and would do better to just stay at home and look after the children, which he has never done before. This woman is not suffering at all from her mother's pressure but would love to continue the symbiosis with her mother with the husband, and so she finds it hard when he is working beyond her range of vision and is not preoccupied with her. She works as a nurse and thus has one foot in contemporary life and another in a traditional culture. Apparently, a daughter can also move on without forming a personal identity and individuality.

We live in a transitional period in which ever more independence is required of women. This can be a struggle that some women find difficult to handle as they continue to feel victimized by their mother. They suppress their anger and cannot free themselves as much as they would like.

Although masochism is not inherent in female development, it does appear quite frequently in women. Problems around separation and sexuality flow together here, as it were. Thus, it is probably a constant that women more readily take on an aggrieved attitude, are more inclined towards a moral (sacrificial) role or sexual masochism and towards depression. Not much has changed in that regard since Electra and the era of antiquity, when women had fewer possibilities for expansion.

Women often suffer from the feeling that they are being tossed between rapprochement and distancing. They cannot free themselves from their mothers without fearing that she will then not love them any longer. Female masochism is thus closely related to problems around separation, notably when the mother–daughter relationship is felt to be oppressive and parasitic. The daughter pays a price for her passive position, which is easily coupled with suffering and submission. In order to win the love of a dismissive mother, the daughter has to put up with all sorts of things. Subsequently, that acquiescence to the mother's wishes is transferred to the husband. Fantasies about playing the whore or being raped by men are therefore not at all rare.

The feeling of self-worth suffers from a lack of independence. In other words, a woman's narcissism suffers from the ambivalent relationship with the mother. A lack of appreciation and a damaged sense of self form a stronger motive than sexuality. However, eroticism can be placed in the service of the sense of self. Women enjoy being flirted with and thus fall into the hands of smooth-talking Don Juans. Love, in the sense of feeling loved, is often a secondary issue for men but holds a central position for women.

Women's masochistic erotic fantasies often find their origin in repressed aggression against the mother. According to Sigmund Freud, this is not true. He assumed that those fantasies were primarily a matter of love for the father. I believe that the fantasies he describes in 'A child is being beaten'[18] are not oedipal fantasies, and I suspect that it is, rather, the mother who is hidden behind the punishing father. Not 'father beats me', but 'I feel I am my mother's attachment and therefore victim' seems to be at the basis of this masturbation fantasy, the way Freud describes it. To be precise, all too often girls feel that they are the extension, the tool, the victim of their (internal) mother (image). The phallic mother, the omnipotent woman in pants whom the girl sees in her imagination, is then replaced by a man. Thus problems of eroticism and aggression, which is what masochism really is, are coupled to each other, and lust through suffering is born.

Women often recount that they let themselves be abused by a man. They complain, but they stay in the relationship nevertheless. It seems incomprehensible but should not be, in light of the prehistory. If a woman has told a wronged and angry story about her lover, I inquire about her relationship with her mother. There then follows an account of the mother that closely resembles the one about her partner – as if the individuals in question had traded places, performing the same role in the same play.

Insofar as masochism plays a role in the development of the woman, and specifically in her relationship with the man, this situation is, in my view, really linked primarily to the original relationship with the mother. When a girl exchanges the mother for the man, when she is chosen without choosing herself, without establishing her independence, she is not a subject of desire. Her desire is then to satisfy the other's desire, and thus she risks becoming tied masochistically to her husband and his desires.

Homosexual longings always continue to play a role for women. Not only can the first husband form a substitute for the first object – the mother – as

Sigmund Freud noted in 1931, but so can the second or third, and he may then be burdened with the legacy thereof.

Generally, the importance of identification with the father is insufficiently recognized in the classic Oedipus complex in relation to girls. Usually girls do not have enough opportunity for identifying with the father as an essential intermediary to be able to arrive at separation from the mother.[19] When her father or mother do not acknowledge the girl as a separate being with her own initiative, the anger that flows from her dependency on the primary object makes an inhibition of open aggression well-nigh inevitable. This repressed anger leads, then, all too easily to victimization and depression.

The role of the father

We know that in the girl's development the father can fulfil a separating function between mother and daughter.[20] In helping the girl not to view the mother as an absolute power any more, he can further her separation. Girls are frequently worried about losing their father's love, since they usually see much less of him. They idealize the father from a distance and long for him. They seek the fulfilment of their heterosexual, erotic, and feminine wishes in their father and later in their husband, which were given no chance with the mother.

The father is also an object of identification, although to a lesser extent. By observing the father and admiring his initiatives, the girl learns to take the lead herself. If she does not want to resemble her mother, it is usually because the latter is too passive, too docile – in short, too masochistic. In that case, the girl prefers to mirror herself in a father who does go his own way.

What you did not get from your mother, you can always try to get from your father. Thus the father fulfils a compensating function in the girl's development. He can make up for something, he can set something straight that she missed in her mother, or what may have been too much of a good thing in the mother. He offers another chance, but one that can also end in a double disappointment.

The girl is also afraid to displease the father, just as she once was afraid to displease her mother. The inhibition of aggression that also plays its part with the father will then make her too docile with him. After all, she hopes to see the idyll that she failed to produce with her mother come to fruition with him. She also tends to idealize her father, because he is less visible and available to her. She tends to give her father credit and demands much less of him than of her mother. Yet he cannot go too far and neglect her too much: in that case she will turn away from him in disappointment and perhaps seek refuge with women instead. Often it is such a double disappointment that is the seed-bed for a lesbian development, much more so than sexual desire.

Girls have a greater tendency towards internalizing relationships: they dream about them, they have all kinds of fantasies about them, which can also make them more vulnerable to disappointments.

In all of this it seems to be more a question of new and different libidinous tendencies directed towards the father rather than one of an object shift. It seems that the mother continues to maintain her old place while the bond with the father is added: he acquires his own place because he has something different to offer. In the course of development nothing is lost: the old is preserved, it is just that something new is always added. In my view, there can be no question of an authentic object shift with regard to the girl – the mother is too important for that, too threatening, and too indispensable.

Obviously, heterosexuality has its say quite early where the father is concerned. Little girls can already be seductive with men and in love with their father. Toddlers who crawl into bed with their parents and push their mother aside show that rivalry between mother and daughter for the father's love begins quite early on. In this sense one could say that the girl separates from the mother earlier than does the boy, who remains in his mother's orbit.[21] The father has something the mother does not, and that gender difference – the deep male voice – is exhilarating and exciting. Women who are crazy about their fathers and do not have a discordant relationship with their mothers often choose men who are the image of their fathers or, at least, resemble him. In that case, we are dealing with a development that is similar to the Oedipus complex of the little boy. The parent of the same gender is then the competitor in acquiring the love of the parent of the opposite gender. The mother remains present in the background as an anchor and will regain a central place at crucial stages in a woman's life, such as during pregnancy and childbirth. Apart from this classic oedipal story, much less has been written on the subject of father and daughter than one might expect, especially in light of the presumed central place of the Oedipus complex in female development.

What does the girl conceal?

'What does woman want?' Up to this point we have encountered three topics in this discussion about which women tend to keep silent. In the first place there is the hatred directed at the mother that must be concealed because the girl cannot do without her for support and refuge. Furthermore, if she hates her mother, with whom she so strongly identifies, then she hates herself as well. This unspoken hate often evokes feelings of guilt. Second, the girl conceals carnal desire and the organ that accompanies it, the clitoris. She has not been taught to name her sexual organs and that, in part, is the reason for her feeling shame around sexual pleasure and the organ that provides it. Third, she remains silent about her yearning for the mother's love because she is embarrassed about the little girl that still lives inside her.

Apart from the fact that women keep silent about their body and their yearnings out of guilt and shame, the silence itself provides an additional reason for shame. The quiet, withdrawn character of many women indicates their insecurity about their place and role. Modesty that is too great can lead to feeling like a minor, and that certainly does not make a woman feel good about herself. This engenders shame about the shame. When speaking and writing are not encouraged socially and stumble upon a taboo inwardly, silence is incorporated in the ego-ideal. This is how the ideal woman should be and behave. It was in protest against this that the English writer Virginia Woolf wrote *A Room of One's Own*[22] early in the twentieth century, at a time when women still had no access to universities and libraries.

In silence, unnoticed, and unconsciously, the girl still longs for her first love object, the mother. Can the most profound longing ever be anything other than finding again the original duality to which the mystic aspires as well[23] and which Sigmund Freud referred to as the oceanic feeling? Is this, perhaps, what woman conceals because she herself does not know?

As I see it, the outlined vicissitudes of development seem to imply over and over again that the mother continues to occupy the primary place in the woman's unconscious. The woman keeps looking for the gratification that the first object provided her with, or withheld from her. As a patient once phrased it concisely: 'I have that longing for my mother, but it is very ambivalent: hold on to me, let me go. It is a matter of attraction and repulsion between us.' In my opinion, in her heart a woman would most like to have a woman with a penis as partner, and because that is not possible, she chooses a man and a bosom (female) friend. In other words, she much prefers to talk with women but is sexually attracted to men.

Woman decoded

Beginning with the earliest phase of child development (the pre-oedipal period), we see that the separation from the omnipotent mother is ambivalent. Not only does the girl want to flee from her dependence on the mother, but she also seeks it, and this lands her in a thorny dilemma. The fears and projections with regard to the mother concern a different fear of castration than in the boy, but a girl is not spared from fear of internal damage or of being broken inside. Serious conflicts with the mother, in particular, lead to the fear of being destroyed by her. The fantasy of being appropriated by the mother, of vanishing inside the mother again, being devoured or broken by her, lead to a reinforced tendency to suppress her own aggression and to premature, excessive adaptation.

In the oedipal phase a girl has to compete with her mother for the father's love. She then sees herself unexpectedly positioned in direct opposition to the love object that, at the same time, is also to offer her protection and security. In this way the Electra complex originates, which is truly complex because of the ambivalent feelings towards the mother. The separation problem of the girl with regard to the mother is repeated in adolescence, while in addition the problem of sexuality needs to be resolved. At that point the normal boy has long reached individuation, gone through separation, and no longer needs to look back.

It makes one wonder if this is the reason why Lot's wife, who looked back at Sodom and Gomorra, was turned into a pillar of salt. After all, a girl automatically falls back into old patterns if she cannot manage to use her aggression for positive goals and mobilize her energy to develop her own initiative. She must engage in a new struggle with the mother, while she feels simultaneously that she is a link in the generational chain and has the image of her own future motherhood in her mind's eye. She must swallow her aggression out of a sense of guilt, which can lead to becoming all too compliant and to remaining immature, or even to masochism and self-destruction.

It seems that the woman is no more capable of an object shift than she is of switching zones by renouncing the clitoris in favour of the vagina. She remains attached to the mother for life, and she seeks in her partner that which she obtained or longed for from, or lacked with, her mother. The girl, in contrast to the boy, lingers in a homosexual object relationship. The desire to shift is certainly present, but loyalty to the original object is too great. If the woman destroys her mother as internal object, it will make her ill, for she is damaging her own image. What I have outlined are primarily the negative, more problematic aspects of female development, the cliffs of which the girl needs to steer clear in order not to remain entangled in an oppressive, infantilizing bond. On the other hand, the bond with the mother is not merely necessary but intimate and growth-promoting as well, precisely because mother and daughter have much in common. However, it is a prerequisite that the mother not only tolerates and allows separation and sexual development, but actually encourages them. When the mother's envy and narcissism do not hamper the girl, if the mother enjoys her own way of functioning and sexual life, she will be able to transfer that to the daughter and will not need her daughter for her personal gratification. In that case, the girl can feel all the more guided and encouraged by her mother. Still, the symbiotic illusion is not cultivated by the mother alone but by the daughter as well. It is a fateful concerted action with two participants.

Among other things, mentioning and naming sexual and physical feelings, functions, and yearnings is important. Positive contact with her own body is not self-evident in girls but is stimulated by the mother, too. In adolescence, particularly, the mother can fulfil an inimitable function by allowing and responding to intimacy, on the one hand, and creating distance and tolerating ambivalence, on the other. In adolescence, girls forcefully repeat the phase of rapprochement of early childhood, which makes a strong appeal to the mother's ability to encourage development. The mother ought to keep a level head when her daughter is capricious and vituperative but wants to crawl onto her lap an hour later. Once again the mother's ability to bear up under the hostility without feeling rejected plays a decisive role.

The girl who is strongly attached to her mother may have the frightening sense that her sexual experience is a burden for her mother. She may imagine that she is failing in her duties towards her mother if she does not make herself wholly available to her.

The feeling that her own pleasure exists at the expense of the other person is easily generalized, and the girl all too often pays for this by abandoning her erotic desires and by feeling forever obligated to her mother. Not only is she responsible for original sin and the expulsion from Paradise because Eve allowed herself to be seduced by the serpent and to eat the forbidden apple, she is also cursed because not only was she denied any pleasure in sex from that time on but, as punishment, God also sentenced her to give birth to her children in pain.

Not only does the woman feel called upon to bear the responsibility for the ups and downs of the children, not only does she have to be a mother who is 'good enough' (an expression of the well-known English paediatrician and psychoanalyst Donald Winnicott), she would actually do well to be better than her own mother.

Chapter 7

Childbirth and depression

The birth of a child can be followed by a psychological disorder in the mother, the gravity and duration of which are variable: everyone is familiar with the passing sadness that comes after giving birth. However, the more persistent neurotic depression is more serious, the collapse of the borderline mother is ominous, and psychosis – the complete loss of any sense of reality after the baby's birth – is life-threatening. The disorder appears as psychosis in 1–3 out of a thousand births, as a serious emotional disorder in 1–3 per cent, as a neurotic depression in 10 per cent, and as a light depression, known as the postpartum blues, supposedly in one out of every three women.[1] These are conservative estimates; the numbers may well be much higher.

Postnatal depression is a universal phenomenon that shows up in every culture; it was described already in antiquity by the physician Hippocrates. However, not until the nineteenth century did psychiatry pay special attention to the topic again, when monographs on the subject appeared in England and France.[2] Since then, psychiatric publications have primarily described symptoms, epidemiology (distribution among the population), and aetiology (cause and history of the origin), but not emotional connections and their significance. For a long time, postnatal depression was explained strictly from the physiological point of view while a psychological explanation failed to appear.

Through the centuries, medical science has assumed all kinds of secretive processes concerning menstruation, pregnancy, birth, and lactation. Postnatal depression was attributed to mysterious events in the woman's body that have always spoken vividly to the imagination. After all, in antiquity it was named 'hysteria' because emotional disorders in women were attributed to a 'roaming' uterus (*hysteros* in Greek). Since the discoveries of endocrinology – the knowledge of internal secretion – in the 1930s, instability after childbirth was generally ascribed to the altered hormonal balance.

However, depression is insufficiently explained as originating in the certainly dramatic physical changes. This is demonstrated, among other things, by the fact that grandmothers and adoptive mothers, too, may have the same symptoms. The birth of a baby disturbs the family's emotional equilibrium.

Feeling supplanted by the baby, the father can also develop complaints that, obviously, have nothing to do with physiology. Furthermore, the psychological changes and adaptations to the new situation are far longer-lasting and more intrusive than the physical ones. Recently, therefore, the tendency has been towards an explanation based on a disturbed psychological and social balance.

In this chapter I discuss the most common form: the non-psychotic variants of postnatal depression. The symptoms vary from rejection of the child to rejection of oneself as mother. In every case it is a matter of regression,[3] a falling back into old patterns of dependency that threatens every new developmental phase in a woman's life, one of which is certainly that of bearing a child. Conflicts around the relationship with the mother's own mother, as I have emphasized, are mentioned by most authors, albeit often not further developed. All sorts of fears can emerge around dependency and wanting to be a baby oneself, feeling like a bad mother, fear around a desire to kill or poison either oneself or the baby, or of being consumed by the baby. The mother experiences great despair, self-reproach, and guilt feelings. Psychosomatic disorders, loss of sexual interest, frequent weeping, anorexia, and hypochondriacal complaints, also with regard to the child, can all be part of it.

Unfortunately, postnatal depression, especially the 'milder' neurotic form that is as frequent as breast cancer, is still a situation that usually escapes the attention of health-care providers. Complaints are rarely treated, unless they result in a full-blown psychosis, which is usually followed by hospitalization and medication without any examination of the background. Prevention of psychological suffering in the subsequent generation and prevention of the present mother's unnecessary suffering ought to motivate the mental health-care professionals to pay greater attention to this problem.[4] Depressed mothers have a disturbing effect on the physical and mental well-being of their baby from the very first day on.

Where psychotherapeutic treatment is concerned, this generally comes about via a psychoanalytic referral. This is why I am surprised that psychoanalysts have not published more on this important subject. One can count on the one hand the number of authors who have pursued these symptoms. Even the psychoanalyst Helene Deutsch, a student of Sigmund Freud's, devotes no more than a few dispassionate phrases on it among her observations on childbirth in her monograph about the psychology of the woman.[5] Extensive case descriptions are lacking, which is the reason why in this chapter I want to delve more deeply into an analysis.

The explanations given in the scanty psychoanalytic literature on postnatal depression follow closely in the footsteps of theoretical changes. The literature of the first half of the twentieth century pays more attention to penis envy, virility complex, castration fear, and woman's masochism and narcissism, in which the baby – following Sigmund Freud – is seen as a substitute for the mother's deficiency. The development of the child's drives is at the centre and takes place in biologically linked phases. The phallic-oedipal phase is of specific importance. The child discovers the constant of gender difference and develops a libidinous bond with the parent of the other gender. Object relationships, the intimate relations of the child with parents or caregivers that are now receiving greater attention, were barely considered at the time. After the Second World War, Anna Freud, Sigmund's daughter, called attention to ego development and defence mechanisms.[6] In addition to the development of the drives, the way in which the drives are controlled by the ego moves forward to become the centre of attention. Even at that time almost nothing was published about postnatal depression.

From the 1960s onward, object relationships, and later on narcissism again, acquire a more central position – the separation between mother and child, the connection with the mother's prehistory, the relationship with the (imaginary) mother, the fantasy significance the child has for her, and, finally, the relationship with the partner and with the child. The followers of Melanie Klein have always paid attention to object relationships, particularly in the sense of fantasies around the internal (imaginary) mothers and fathers. The 'splitting' into 'good' and 'bad' objects that accompany these, the various projections and projective identifications as concepts, are quite useful in studying the preoccupations of the mother with regard to her child and her mother, as the following will clarify.

All the viewpoints mentioned, supplemented by more recent insights, are applicable to Anitra, the woman to be discussed next. Two aspects that I worked out previously concerning disorders in the mother–daughter relationship can be tested here for their applicability: first of all, the multi-generational involvement and, second, the symbiotic illusion. Postnatal depression is pre-eminently a disorder that has to do with the mother–daughter relationship. The two families – the one to which the mother belongs and the one she herself starts – become connected to each other and so form a link in the generational chain. Thus it is remarkable how often the mother's mother herself had also suffered from postnatal depression and how this episode sometimes returns at the time that her daughter gives birth, as was the case here as well.

Being depressed after a birth is not always accompanied by an unequivocal rejection of the child. A disorder may manifest itself in the mother's attachment to her child, but not always. In fact, it often affects specifically good and caring mothers, although the ambivalence and the tendency to deny this are always rather great. Sometimes the rejection of the child is at the core of the depression, sometimes it is more a question of despair, helplessness, the sense of failing the child – even when the child is doing fine, as was the case with Anitra. Here the image of the woman with anorexia nervosa comes to mind, for in that case, too, the girl is absolutely convinced that she is fat, even though this does not correspond to reality. Similarly, a woman who has just given birth can feel worried and laden with guilt: no matter how hard she tries, it is never enough. Even if she watches over the child around the clock, she continues to feel that she is remiss in her duties.

Anitra

Anitra appears for our first conversation with a can of milk powder – not by accident, as it will turn out later. Fantasies around devouring, being devoured, starvation, and being poisoned are central to her perception. It strikes me that Anitra looks rather unhealthy: she is a bit shabby and some- what boyishly dressed, and has a very troubled look in her eyes. She lets it be known that she has come with very mixed feelings, is really quite reluctant, although at the same time she is also very friendly and well-disposed.

Her story is full of contradictions: actually there 'isn't anything really wrong with me', although she goes around weeping all day long and con- stantly picks arguments with her partner. This began after the birth of their first, unplanned, and completely unexpected child. Anitra is close to 40 years old and has never really wanted any children. She is opposed to the role of women in our society and now feels entirely at the mercy of her fate: circum- stances have forced her to be the slave of her partner and her child.

She is deeply shocked by a fantasy of throwing her child out of the window; she is equally afraid of poisoning the baby boy with her breast milk, and she feels very guilty about these and other, similar thoughts.

She recounts that she enjoyed a childhood without any serious problems and that the relationship with her parents is a good one. However, her mother showed no reaction to the announcement that her daughter was pregnant, nor does she show any interest in the baby now. It seems to Anitra as if she would rather not touch him.

Anitra has always suffered from serious headaches, especially during menstruation (this happens frequently in the case of women with postnatal depression and probably has to do with anger about, and partly rejection of, the woman's role or the female sexual identity), but she is convinced that this is a purely physical phenomenon. To her surprise, she enjoyed being preg- nant; it was the first time that she felt like super-woman and mother when she was waddling around with her big belly. The shock was therefore all the greater once the child was born and she felt empty, flat, and destitute. She missed carrying the child and felt great nostalgia for the pregnancy: a clearly female reaction.

Since the birth, Anitra is furious with her boyfriend, who, she assumes, will not help and support her. She feels utterly abandoned by him, although she has to admit that he actually does a lot for her and tries to come to her aid wholeheartedly. Initially, she was angry with the child as well, who demanded so much of her and so entirely changed her life. I have the impression that she thinks she must now lead the female life that in her eyes was so contemptible and that she had always managed to avoid before. She continued working after the baby was born, but that, too, has suddenly become too cumbersome.

Her account shows that Anitra is a true perfectionist who wants to arrange everything for everyone else to the last detail, while she tends to neglect herself.

Although psychoanalysis appears threatening to her, Anitra goes along with it. Even though she is desperate, she maintains that there is nothing wrong with her. My impression is that the regression, the setback in competence, the dependency, the admission of weakness that for her goes hand in hand with analysis, are a fearful spectre. From the very first moment on, the conflicts of ambivalence – familiar from the literature – revealed themselves, and to me as her psychoanalyst as well. Needing someone implies imperfection and therefore failure, it seems.

It soon becomes clear that Anitra definitely has a problematic background and comes from a discordant family. In the first place, her mother lost her own mother at a very young age: she was only 3 years old, and the circumstances were dramatic. Her mother's mother died in the Indonesian jungle – it is presumed not from starvation but from overeating. The story, which seems partly symbolic and should probably be attributed to family mythology, obviously contains a kernel of truth as well. Once more it has to do with the theme of eating, which had already played an important role for the grandmother. Furthermore, I am now encountering an ever-recurring fantasy about life and death that in the past, sadly, has been definitely based on reality – namely, that when there is one who arrives, there is one who must depart. When a child arrives, a mother dies, or, vice versa, the child must be killed before it devours the mother.

The little girl that Anitra's mother then was suffered desperately. Not only had she lost her mother, but she subsequently led a nomadic existence. She was lodged with a foster family or was roaming through the jungle on horseback, alone with her father, who was an adventurer. It is not hard to predict what will happen when this emotionally neglected girl eventually starts her own family. The problems will continue to have their effect on several more generations.

All of this shows why Anitra's mother was terrified of having children, which is hardly surprising after what she and her own mother had been through. When she was pregnant with Anitra, she became panic-stricken and had serious hypochondriacal complaints. She suffered ferocious abdominal pains and elected to have surgery for an alleged appendicitis. The ensuing course of events leads to my supposition that she was thereby having a symbolic abortion. However, it failed; she had two children in rapid succession whom she did not want, and, as Anitra later recounted, she felt absolutely devastated.

When Anitra was a toddler, her step-grandmother died. This grandmother had come to live with Anitra's parents when she was ill, and her stepdaughter thereupon cared for her as if she were her own mother. Thus, just as in Anitra's own case, there were demands on her mother from two sides. Anitra's mother had to take care of a mother and of a child at the same time, which was clearly too much for her.

Only gradually did I come to realize that Anitra's mother herself must have suffered from postnatal depression at the time. Her ambivalence, her mixed feelings for her (step)mother and for her child seem suspiciously similar to the emotions with which Anitra is struggling now. Insofar as I am able to reconstruct the situation, this depression seems to have been initiated by the memory of her mother's death when she was small and actualized by the death of her stepmother. It seems that at Anitra's birth there was a question of a split as well as a reversal: the anger at the mother was directed at the baby (Anitra), while the positive feelings went to the stepmother whose caretaker Anitra's mother was at that time, thus offering what she herself had not received.

Anitra, who, according to her mother, was a skinny and ugly baby, developed an eating disorder. Her mother's negative feelings had led to the baby's early weaning after a breast infection, as a result of which she was given food that she was unable to digest. The baby might have felt she was poisoned by her mother. Freud wrote in 1933: '... we discover *the fear of being murdered or poisoned*, which may later form the core of a paranoic illness, already present in this pre-oedipal period, *in relation to the mother*' (italics added).[7] She became so emaciated and dehydrated that they feared for her life; after being hospitalized, she was finally put on a diet of beans. Presumably she was allergic to cow's milk and therefore it was difficult to feed her. Thus, as a baby, Anitra was actually starving. The approach to this problem seems rather Spartan or, indeed, nineteenth-century to me.

Allegedly Anitra was an extremely difficult and demanding toddler, who cried constantly and followed her mother everywhere. The latter could not even go to the bathroom in peace because, to her great irritation, the child would keep banging on the door until she reappeared. Because her step-mother was then near death in her home, she had no time for her child. Almost 40 years later, Anitra still had to listen to these tales and was after all that time still expected to feel sorry for her mother. Her mother thought that having children was such a great catastrophe, and she had been so exhausted and ill that after the birth of her second daughter she had herself secretly sterilized, although her husband would have liked a son. Everything points to the fact that Anitra's mother wants attention to be paid to her struggle with her past and now desires additional maternal care from her daughter.

Anitra, who has always been a loyal, docile, caring daughter, cannot muster all of this now that she has her own child. These stories induce a silent and controlled powerful storm in her, and she begins to hate her mother more and more. Instead of the support that she hoped for now that she herself is a mother, all she hears is that in reality she herself did not have a mother either.

Over and above this, her mother develops all sorts of hypochondriacal complaints during the first year of her grandson's life, so that Anitra begins to fear for her mother's life although the doctors cannot find anything wrong with her.

It seems that the mother is opening every valve in order not to lose her daughter's attention. She always fully agreed with her daughter's wish not to have children, and now she feels betrayed. The arrival of the grandchild as a rival is a true disaster for her. The loss of, and the mourning for, her own mother are concretized and symbolized by the 'loss' of her daughter whom in later years she had begun to consider as a mother. Furthermore, her jealousy of the baby that she herself wants to be all the more vehemently revives her need for a mother. In short, after her daughter's delivery Anitra's mother seems to be going through a repetition of her own postnatal depression. In addition, the narrative reveals the intensity of her mother's life course to such an extent that it seems as if Anitra has identified with it.

After her traumatic infancy and early childhood, Anitra went through a dramatic change when the ugly duckling grew into the well-behaved model child. Her younger sister, who had been a 'beautiful and good' baby, grew into the nuisance in the household; she always succeeded in driving her father into a fury, and he, to some extent, then vented his anger at his wife on Anitra's sister. He was constantly watching his younger daughter, who should have been the son he had wanted, and he always had something critical to say, whereupon all hell would break loose again. Anitra was the easygoing, successful child, a fast learner and good at sports. She did her utmost to keep the peace in the house at any cost, distracted the others, and attempted to change the subject when things became controversial. In addition, she did her best to be the athletic son her father did not have.

Anitra's mother was the martyr in the family – the father's drudge and slave. He would always make angry scenes, usually around trivia having to do with eating – with the table manners of the 'faulty' daughter or with the salt and pepper that were missing from the table. Out of fear of her tyrannical husband, the mother would then wear herself out trying to make up for it. Father settled half-heartedly for his oldest daughter as the substitute son, just as long as she achieved. To this day he pounds her on the shoulder when greeting her, warmly but roughly, as men are wont to do with each other, almost as if he wants to knight her symbolically. He would also have much preferred for his daughter's child to bear his last name, apparently considering the boy as his own son and thereby suggesting an incestuous situation.

Anitra has always had a clandestine understanding with her mother in that she listened to her poisonous complaints about her husband. At such times the mother is identifying with her daughter, suggesting that they are having exactly the same experiences with those dreadful men in their lives. According to Anitra, her mother does not listen to her at all but speaks only about herself, constantly asking for advice and support but not listening to the answers and never following up on them. She refuses to hear anything that does not agree with her own definition of the situation, which is that they are both victims. Anitra feels herself totally dissolving in this request for attention where her own identity does not matter: she melts into her needy mother, as it were, something she experiences as a serious threat.

In the transference I recognize what Anitra recounts about the interaction between herself and her mother. With me, she fulfils the position that her mother holds with regard to her: she complains, she asks for advice, and she will not accept what I say. Consequently, I can readily imagine her irritation. She can never stop talking about her husband and women friends, all of whom lean on her but give nothing in return, and thus she is the victim. At the same time, she rejects the help she asks for, which has an undermining effect.

She has a great deal of trouble entrusting her child to her partner or to anyone else. She finds inappropriate caretakers who, according to her, then do not do things right, so that she really cannot go to work or come to me. She makes no comments or criticisms but is silently furious, she weeps with misery and frustration and practically chokes on her sense of being wronged and on her powerlessness. She is never at peace and knows only how to sacrifice herself. The relationship with her partner is bad, and mutual undercutting is the order of the day there as well.

I use the way I experience the situation – as she succeeds in evoking it in me without ever directly involving me in anything verbally – to clarify to her what she is doing with me. She is unconsciously trying to elicit a position from me that demonstrates a strong analogy with what her mother does to her. I use the countertransference, making myself aware of my own emotional reactions – an irreplaceable resource – to discover what is actually the matter between Anitra and her mother. This consultation of the experience that a patient incites in the analyst is crucial and is certainly valid in the case of this woman, who has such difficulty in separating truth from fiction. She has little interest in the space between individuals, the virtual; that which might be played out between us is not something she wants to examine. She is not exactly sure what it is she wants from me or what she has against me. The one thing Anitra is very sure of is that she feels nothing special for me and has no desire to become personal with me. Her thinking is black and white, all or nothing. She does not need me and apparently comes only because I think it is necessary. I am the expert, nothing more; she does not miss me on weekends or during vacations. In a nutshell, insofar as she is aware, she has no meaningful feeling whatsoever where I am concerned. No feelings of transference are verbalized, her understanding of her own inner world has to be built up from scratch.

Gradually it becomes clear to her how her interplay with her mother works and what her inner mother image looks like: someone who, she feels, fails her immeasurably. Instead of a mother and a daughter, an adult and a child, the roles have become reversed: the wisest had to be the oldest. Now, in its place, a situation has been created where Anitra and her mother have both become babies and are competing with the real baby. During the analysis there is a fairly rapid breakthrough of this pattern because Anitra becomes aware of her anger at and her disappointment in her mother. Against her better judgment, she no longer tries to maintain the symbiotic illusion with the mother by giving her what she had wanted to receive herself. She gambles with the domestic peace and withdraws increasingly from the role of being her mother's caretaker. She takes more pleasure in directing her attention to her son, notices that she actually likes having a child, and is even able to enjoy it.

In addition to a renewed connection with her father, all sorts of other shifts are taking place as well. Anitra develops splits similar to those that ruled the family before. In the first place, she and her sister had been split into the 'good' and 'bad' daughter. Now she is splitting the 'bad' mother–baby and the 'good' real baby, while she begins to see the 'good' man in her son and the 'bad' one in her partner. Her father is given the more oedipal role because she is finally giving him the son he had always wanted, and so he has a less ambivalent attitude to her as a woman. Of course, this is fostered because the father's access to the daughter becomes possible only now that the symbiotic illusion with the mother has been interrupted by the birth of a son: Anitra triumphs in the rivalry with her mother. She has a sense of having accomplished more, she has provided her father with that which her mother was unable to provide. He brings her flowers and is proud of her.

On the other hand, Anitra begins to be more like her mother now, which is exactly what women such as she fear: to be thrown back on their own mother with every new phase of life – the mother whom they do not want to resemble, of whom they are afraid, with whom they do not want to identify, on whom they do not want to be dependent again. Inadvertently, Anitra is experiencing a strong identification with her mother, whose life she has to repeat, as it were: just like her mother, she suffers from depression and feels a tendency to want to get rid of her child. When the feelings around mother and child have to some extent been worked through, the conflict is repeated in a different form: she now has an almost irresistible inclination to throw her partner out. The only feeling she has left for him any longer is hate. Furthermore, the problem manifests itself throughout the analysis in the transference: Anitra constantly wants to push me away and get rid of me as her analyst.

The sadness and emotional pain caused by the lack of a loving mother lasts for the entire analysis – the anger is extensively worked through. Still, she is not well equipped to admit her longings to herself, and certainly not to admit that she is settling in with me. During every holiday period she is allegedly happy to have the analysis interrupted; she never misses me and often looks for an excuse to terminate the analysis prematurely. She tends to live her need for my help and support through projective identification – that is to say, by placing it in others and taking care of them. That is also what her army of needy women friends are for, who come to her to complain and cry on her shoulder. She always listens patiently to everything without ever saying a word about herself. Although she does feel victimized by these egocentric women friends who never ask about her, she maintains that she has nothing to complain about or any right to do so – after all, they are much worse off than she is. In actuality, she herself has become a 'therapist' and denies her unmistakable role as patient with me, which makes my persona all the more intolerable to her, even though it is quite noticeable that she is also rather fond of me.

I often find her lively way of thinking original and captivating; she expresses herself precisely and well and, despite everything, attends her sessions faithfully. She continues to complain that she needs love and attention and would so much like to have her partner help her. I do not believe she herself is aware of her exacting demands – rather, she is under the impression that she must constantly comply with the wishes of others. In the meantime, she is demanding and insatiable when not all of her demands are met. This could be the greediness of the oral phase, a regression to the infant stage to which the literature about postpartum depressions often refers. She is angry but has trouble expressing her anger. She makes herself elusive, for her resistance is quite indirect. She presents herself as slavish and subservient, but surreptitiously she wrecks everything I offer while noisily lamenting her fate. She is incapable of accepting any help, above all from her analyst, whom she envies. Other than meekly admiring the fact 'that I am always there for her', she rarely or never has any associations that refer to me.

Her fear of dependency and her need for control are expressed in another way as well: she speaks compulsively, thematically, without a trace of any free association, and thereby she beats any subject she introduces to death. Dreams or fantasies are rarely brought up, although from time to time she does actually have a very animated dream or fantasy that helps us to clarify that which unconsciously preoccupies her. Her conscious experience is astonishing in its magical colouring – in other words, thoughts are the equivalent of facts and concrete events.

The roles are skilfully reversed. As the analyst, I am turned into the powerless toddler, pointlessly banging on the emotional door that mother keeps hermetically sealed. The link with the prehistory on the mother's side becomes most obvious in the fixation on food, nursing, and poisoning. Anitra is afraid she will poison her child via the cancer and 'shit' that her women friends pour out over her. She argues perpetually with her partner about food that, she claims, has been in the refrigerator too long. He always wants to save everything because it can still be used, even after the expiration date has passed, while she wants to throw everything out because it has turned into poison. She does not interpret that thought as a fantasy but as a menacing fact.

One time she impulsively rips a laburnum out of the ground (putting it in the street as a 'foundling' so that a pedestrian will find and adopt it and the plant can thus survive anyway) because its seed is poisonous. She is afraid her child will sit down under the tree and die from eating the 'poisonous seed'. The analogies impose themselves here: the grandmother who was poisoned by food, her life that is poisoned by her demanding, ungenerous mother, and her partner who impregnated her with his poisonous semen. She is pre-occupied with health food and alternative, especially oral, medications. Milk and meat are basically wicked.

When Anitra turns out to be pregnant a second time – unexpectedly, as she claims, accidentally on purpose – she grows even more hostile with regard to her environment and me. She is afraid I will hamper her independence and she fears my disapproval. I am replacing the jealous mother. She is also afraid that the older child will choke on his jealousy, and she dreams that he dies, devoured by a crocodile. When one child arrives, another must depart – a symbol to which Anitra gives concrete expression by naming the child after the drowned child of a friend. She absolutely does not want a girl: she can't 'make her into a woman'. Her fantasy goes haywire at the thought of a baby girl. She thinks in that case her mother will die and come back in the form of the baby girl, or that the child will die, that she will kill it, and so on. I believe that a girl would aggravate her fear of her own baby yearnings and would make her more jealous of the baby.

It is at this time that Anitra's son has his first asthma attacks. She more or less accuses the doctors of trying to kill him and always calls for medical help at the very last moment. Once again she feels terribly pressured from all sides. She wants to quit analysis. For a variety of reasons she cannot abide me any longer. On the one hand, she is afraid that I will be a leech on her, just like her mother, that she will have to take care of me by taking me into account, while she already has plenty to do with two children. On the other hand, I need to be removed because of the renewed threat of her becoming too dependent on me.

Thus Anitra declares that she wishes to terminate her analysis after the birth of her second child. I see this decision as premature and inspired by fear. She could very well suffer a second postnatal depression, as she is still quite unstable. In addition, I have the sense that her anger and bloodthirsti-ness against her mother are landing in my lap. That is fine, but not if she wants to 'abort' me, as it were, as the unwanted child, as her mother did. If I am the unwanted baby girl, I am her problem, and that would in no way elucidate and resolve her confusion. But, since Anitra leaves no room for symbolism, she turns her imagined hostility into concrete action. Her ambivalence is enormous and insurmountable. In her inner theatre the nega-tive and positive emotional currents are each given a way out. She functions on a dream level following her unrealistic fantasies instead of being con-nected to reality. In addition to doing me in, if she leaves, she will rescue me from her destructive tendencies. Furthermore she will rescue herself, the child, and her mother: nothing can happen to them when I as witch am sacrificed in their place. At least, she cannot be thrown out any more, and neither can her child, who is not welcome, should it be a girl. The analyst seems to represent the female baby she once was and that her mother and now she, too, do not want to have. Moreover, by separating – that is, by rejecting the 'unwanted' mother she projects onto me – Anitra can maintain the contact with her real mother.

Looking back, it is dramatic how after the birth of her child Anitra no longer knows how to handle her female role. The equilibrium has been disrupted because she has to be lover, breadwinner, mother, and daughter all at the same time. She compensates for her increased vulnerability after childbirth by dominating her partner more while she, quite paradoxically, at the same time masks this by masochistically playing at being his victim. She is somewhat compulsive and has a hard time summoning the psychological flexibility that the birth of a child requires to find a new emotional balance. She tends to solve everything by projection, projective identification, and splitting, but under the changed circumstances these mechanisms no longer suffice.

To this mother the normal regression to the 'primary maternal preoccupation'[8] – as Winnicott describes the emotional situation of a young mother – is a threat. She will look to the more active approach of perfectionism in caring for her child. This tires her out, and she becomes desperate, slipping into a depression. Denying the seriousness of the situation – also well known from the literature – is clearly recognizable. There can be no question of falling back on the mother, for which every woman longs during the delivery period, because of (internal) conflicts with her. This, too, is characteristic. No support can be expected from Anitra's mother. The reverse is more likely: her mother seeks support from her. This makes her even angrier and more desperate, while at the same feeling guilty towards her mother.

Something else is at play: in postnatal depression the young mother often has the fantasy that she has taken the child from her mother, that the mother will become jealous and take the child back. Rivalry between mother and daughter frequently resumes around the birth of a child. The thinking then is: my mother will begrudge me the child, I may not become a mother for then my mother will be jealous, she is the only one with the right to have children, and so forth. All of this results in the daughter feeling pursued by the mother's envy. In Anitra the rivalry with the mother and the renewed oedipal bond with the father are clearly identifiable.

The jealousy of the partner who threatens to be pushed into the background so that the baby will be hers alone also indicates the rivalry with men. Because she did not suffice as a woman, she will now prove that she can handle things alone. She divides her anger: her son becomes her idol, for he is a part of her and is what she had wanted to be. While her mother and her partner are cast as the 'bad guys', he is the 'good', the fantastic son. This gives her the chance to take pleasure in him, and she does take care of him in exemplary fashion. Yet, he continues to be at the centre of the altercations between his parents, and within the year, when Anitra has accidentally become pregnant again, he develops a serious case of bronchial asthma. This may be caused in part by the fact that the mother's ambivalence behind all her good care is tangible to the child.

After the birth of Anitra's first child, whom she had unexpectedly at a later age, huge shifts take place in the two families, her mother's and her own. Everyone threatens to become jealous of everyone else. Anitra is jealous of her partner because he has her take care of the baby while he is free to come and go. Her mother is jealous of the baby that she wants to be herself, and of Anitra because she has a son. Anitra's partner is jealous of her because she will not let him near the child, and of the baby who gets the love that she withholds from him. Anitra's father is jealous of her partner because he is a rival who, to top it all off, sired a son.

And this is not all. Throughout her life Anitra has had serious conflicts around activity versus passivity, male versus female identity, masochism versus sadism, eating versus being eaten, poisoning versus being poisoned, killing versus being killed. All of this is reinforced by the weakening of the defence mechanisms that take place around childbirth in the woman's inner world. Fortunately the treatment, and perhaps its termination, have made it possible for her to feel more self-reliant and in charge of her own body. In any event, after the birth of the second child there was no new postnatal depression.

In a follow-up contact it turns out that Anitra and her family are doing well. The problems did not arise again, the oldest child's asthma has disappeared, and she speaks more warmly about her relationship with her partner.

Together with the unresolved symbiosis with the mother, a tragic lack of maternal care two generations earlier – and who knows how many times before that – led to a 'symbiotic disillusion'. Anitra became profoundly disappointed that the strong bond she thought she had with her mother was based on nothing more than a small alliance against her father. When her daughter is pregnant, the mother fails her. The symbiosis with the mother has been thoroughly disrupted by reality. The subsequent depression originates in a whole series of changes and shifts. First, in the mourning around the 'loss' of the child: Anitra experienced the separation at birth very dramatically. She lost the symbiosis with the foetus that in her fantasy represented the fiercely longed-for duality between mother and child.

Mother–daughter symbiosis and postnatal depression after delivery

To some extent my two hypotheses about the symbiotic illusion and the multi-generation transmission along the female line overlap. In postnatal depression the mother–daughter relationship is of very specific importance. The mother who has herself not had a satisfactory relationship with her mother tends to lean on her daughter. Usually this problem goes back several generations, and we see a failed separation along the female line, transmitted from mother to daughter.

In unsatisfactory mother–child relationships a mixture of super-involvement and inadequate contact tend to go hand in hand with moments of overindulgence and neglect. The mother can easily fixate on a daughter whom she unconsciously confuses with the mother image for which she longs so intensely, so that the child becomes her mother's therapist. Consequently, in such cases on the one hand the daughter has always been overburdened, and on the other she has trouble freeing herself from the symbiosis with the mother. She will be inclined to recoil from pregnancy. If she then has a child after all, the fact that she herself never had a real childhood will be emphasized more strongly. She will feel overburdened because she has already had to continually support and sustain her mother, and now there is the addition of a real child. Her envy of the baby will be all the greater because of it, especially because around childbirth a reinforced, frightening oral regression shows up in the mother. In part she identifies with her baby. The young mother does not want to be merely a mother, she wants to be the baby who is being cared for at the same time.

Her ambivalence increases all the time, and with it so does her despair. She hates the child because once again it requires her to take care of it instead of being cared for herself. The magic bond of the symbiotic illusion, which existed between the mother and daughter, seems to have been acutely disrupted at the birth of the baby. Both the mother and the daughter sense the other as being 'unfaithful'. The hostility that was always repressed and concealed by the symbiotic idyll – the holding onto and idealizing of one another – now threatens to explode in full force. The hatred, successfully repressed up to that point, threatens to be discharged via splitting onto the child, particularly if it is a girl. The old conflict – that the dependency on and the anger against the mother are highly incompatible – returns in all its strength.

Furthermore, during the childbirth period the woman feels threatened by the intensifying identification with her mother, an identification that raises a spectre for her as well. The ambivalence conflict, expressed in the fear of separation with regard to the internal image of the mother and the yearning for an idyllic or oceanic union with her, leads to depression after childbirth, which is experienced as a loss of the dyad.

In every case the formation of a new family signifies a critical situation that can easily end in a crisis. Pregnancy is a time of regression, delivery is a time of separation, and the concern and care-giving mean that one's own interests must be partly abandoned. It is self-evident that the child inspires love, but hatred as well. The repressed anger at the child, the sadness and mourning for one's own lost childhood, the missed chances, the problems that a woman can encounter in her role as mother, may all surface in great turbulence.

The child infringes on the relationship between the parents: with this new responsibility it is more difficult for them to remain children, they move up as a generation. They identify with the baby and its privileges but are also jealous of them. The father feels excluded from the mother's intimacy with the child and turns into the jealous older brother, as it were, who now has to be an adult. The mother longs for her own infancy, for her own mother, she wants more of what she enjoyed at that time or wants to recover what she missed.

The mother's falling back onto her own mother can remain an unfulfilled longing. It can also lead, to the previously mentioned mother phobia, to aversion: mother may not come near, she may not touch the child, she may not meddle in any way. These feelings originate during the childbirth period from the fear of regressing to a dependent or longing position with regard to one's own mother – in short, from the fear of becoming a baby oneself again.

Not only can the bond with the mother be reinforced through delivering a baby, but the same is also true for the oedipal bond with the father. The new mother feels like her father's child again, she wants to push her mother aside and have her father to herself. Even the desire to have his child emerges again in her revived, unconscious child's fantasy. She can still develop the feeling of really being married to her father, while her husband may matter less. Devaluing the partner and claiming the child for herself alone has serious consequences, among other things for the psycho-sexual development of the child. Gender identity in boys suffers from a bond with the mother that is too close. For girls the consequences are less drastic, and yet, not being released from the childhood bond with the mother is an impediment to their own development, too.

A 30-year-old woman, who had been in treatment with me as a child, recently returned because she was having problems. For the past ten years she has had a much older male partner, but there is no sexual relationship. She sleeps with him in one bed the same way she used to sleep with her single mother before. She never freed herself from the mother enough to enter into a satisfactory relationship with a man. The agonizing and unresolved homosexual bond – in the looser sense of the word – with the mother often leaves no room for a genuine relationship with anyone else.

In order to answer the question whether pathology will or will not be transmitted to successive generations, it is of overriding importance that forming a new family go hand in hand with the release of the childhood bonds with the parents and the family of origin. The new mother must have gone through the separation of her internal mother image and individuation to some extent, at least, so as not to look for similarities with her mother in her husband or to hate her mother in him. She must have brought the oedipal relationship with her father to a positive end in order not see her child as her father's child. In turn, the grandparents are faced with the task once again of withdrawing from the oedipal bonds with their children and making space for a new generation and a new family. All of these demands cannot always be met, so that postnatal depression is a fairly common phenomenon.

Because of the woman's suffering and because of the prevention pertaining to the child as well, it is extremely important that postnatal depression be treated. Postnatal depression is unfortunately an ill-served subject, not only in practice but in psychoanalytic theory, too, in part because mothers receive little attention since they are usually considered from the child's viewpoint. However, the young child's disorder cannot be understood without including the mother's fantasy in the process. What must be considered are the longings, ideals, and fears that the mother attempts to realize via the child and in what way she therein feels frustrated, pursued, and threatened by the child. In other words, the question is to what extent the mother projects the characteristics she so intensely yearns for onto the child in order to complete herself that way, and to what extent she attributes aggression and maligned characteristics (projective identification) to the child, whereupon she will feel threatened by these.

Usually, postnatal depression can be treated quite successfully and is often quickly resolved. The perinatal period is such a far-reaching upheaval that the overall sensitivity to outside influences and the need for change are greater than normal. All gates are still open, as it were, making women more accessible in this phase of their life.

Chapter 8

Martha

A woman in her middle years

The middle years of life, besides bringing a deterioration of the vital functions, can also be grounds for renewed progress, development, and creativity. Facing finiteness and mortality can increase and intensify the quality of subjective experience, provided that mourning over what has been lost and the fear of death can be sufficiently worked through.[1]

Particularly in the life of women, significant changes can come about in this middle phase, both professionally and privately. Obviously, there are differences between women who have both an active professional life and a family, women who do not work but do have children, and those who have never been parents.

This chapter deals chiefly with the first group of women, and most specifically with their experiences during the period after the children have left home. It is self-evident that at this stage parents will be confronted more intensely than before with the scope and content of their partnership and that their mutual relationship will therefore take a more central position than was previously the case.

On the basis of the case description of an analysand whom I shall call Martha, several theoretical viewpoints regarding the middle years will be clarified. Based on her account, various matters will come up for discussion. To what extent is Martha's development during the middle years connected to aspects of the mother–daughter relationship when observed across three generations (Martha's mother, Martha herself, Martha's daughter)? Earlier chapters dealt primarily with the neurotic aspects of the mother–daughter relationship that impede or cause stagnation in the emotional development. At this time, in contrast, I want to emphasize the healthy sides and hope to call attention to the progressive and growth-inciting tendencies in the relationship between mother and daughter.

Thus, the concern is not with a case history or the course of a given treatment, but is merely the follow-up of a previous, fairly successful psychoanalysis. We shall show the positive after-effects that resulted from the treatment, as well as the problems that remained unresolved. The assumption is that Martha's treatment had a favourable influence on her further

development during the middle years. However, we also know from the literature that treatment during the years of childhood, puberty, or adolescence –
as was the case here – is, unfortunately, no guarantee for the formation
of psychological problems in subsequent phases of life. These data are
confirmed by Martha's history.

Martha's life story

Martha is around 50 years old when she returns to me, her former analyst,
for a number of discussions about her current situation. This offers me
the opportunity not only to hear directly from her how she has fared since
the analysis, but also – with her full consent – to use the material for my
argument.

Martha is already well into the experience of what used to be called 'middle
age', which is now more optimistically known as the middle years. Not only
has she acquitted herself of the responsibility of raising her children to her
own satisfaction, she has also – after long hesitation because of the children –
made the 'painful' decision, as she puts it, of leaving her husband and ending
her marriage of 25 years. After some difficult years (further discussed below)
she has managed to find again her sense of self-esteem and balance. There is
room for entering into a new relationship and for continued development of
her creativity.

Martha had started her first analysis because she was suffering from bouts
of depression. In addition, she always recoiled from lasting relationships
while, at the same time, wanting them as well. She longed for a partner and
for children. However, her fear of commitment led to relationships with
married men or with men whom she could handle easily but who, for that
same reason, did not really enthral her. She had lost her father when she was
quite young, and since then she had already gone through a number of relationships with older men. Thus, seen superficially, for her it was a matter of
missing the beloved father (oedipal issues).

However, it was the analysis that first showed that Martha had separated
very little from her first object, her mother. In her experience this mother
image was still quite omnipotent. Moreover, her mother had been seriously
traumatizing for Martha in her childhood years, not merely in her fantasy
but in reality as well. The mother had neglected her, was aggressively out of
control, frenzied, mistrustful. In addition, linked to her mistrust, she reacted
by being highly restrictive and controlling. Martha had always felt her
mother's moods, explosions, and rage to be extremely threatening.

Embarking on a course to bring the unresolved negative relationship with
her mother to a good end, seeing a female analyst seemed to offer the best
chance for success. Viewed in retrospect, the negative transference did not
come adequately into its own at the time. Nevertheless, progress was made in
this analysis, and new development moved forward.

After some five years of treatment, and with mutual agreement, Martha wanted to terminate the analysis. She was in love with a man her own age and her equal, whom she subsequently married.

Martha and her husband had three children, two sons and then a daughter, all of whom are now more or less grown up. She states that, although problematic, the marriage seemed quite solid at first. There was the period of creating family and raising children, which left little room for paying attention to each other and for the difficulties in the relationship. Gradually, however, a joint sadomasochistic game between the partners developed, growing ever tighter, in which Martha felt herself to be the increasingly neglected victim.

Thanks to self-analysis and self-insight, in part the result of her psychoanalytic treatment, Martha managed to recognize her situation. She decided that she no longer wanted to play a masochistic role, which she had viewed as inescapable when the children were small. At that time she would put up with anything to save her marriage. Now, however, she noticed more and more that she felt invariably lonely in her husband's company.

For a long time she kept trying to improve the unsatisfactory relationship. An attempt at couples' therapy was bumpy and did not produce any true progress. Martha felt with growing clarity that the more she struggled to get out of her desperate plight, the more her husband's hostility increased. In the end, she realized that it was pointless to continue the relationship this way. She suggested separation, which was soon followed by divorce.

Martha at middle age

Initially Martha lived through a period of great social fear and uncertainty. In her own eyes she often did not know what her attitude towards the outside world should be, and she felt as if she barely knew where she stood any more. These feelings were closely tied to her changed social status after the divorce. She had the frightening sensation that she suddenly had to face life without a man's protection. As she prepared for the big step, she had weighed the advantages more heavily than the risks. The gain of independence had been a sharper image for her than the loss – the sadness – that the dissolution of her marriage also brought with it. What mattered in the end, however, was that she had regained her freedom. Once again, she was an independent woman, standing on her own feet, as before. Yet there was an important difference from that earlier time, whose instinctive consequences she had not sufficiently considered beforehand either: she was now beyond the menopause and no longer the blooming young girl of earlier days.

Nevertheless, Martha gradually regained a certain sense of self-worth. She developed enough self-confidence to renew old friendships and start in on new connections as well, both in her private life and in her work environment. To her pleasure, she discovered that she had greater creative possibilities in her professional life than before, if only because she now had more time and opportunity to shape her scientific interests.

This situation is consistent with what the psychoanalyst Erik H. Erikson, Anna Freud's contemporary, and others assert about the 'middle years': not only do loving bonds become more important, but work does as well.[2] Among other things, the professional experience gained can generate extremely productive years. Accordingly, after her divorce Martha took greater pleasure in her profession as a university instructor. She organized her life as a single woman, had frequent contact with women friends, and did not expect ever to enter into a new relationship again.

Martha in love

Nevertheless, a few years later Martha moved her life in a different direction. To her own surprise, she not only 'fell spontaneously in love for the first time in her life' – her own words – but these feelings appeared to be mutual. Both felt they had found a suitable life partner, especially on an emotional level, albeit late in life. They discovered that previously they had each looked for support in a partner who gave priority to order and common sense and thus formed their strict, reprimanding polar opposite. Now that the building phase of their life was definitively behind them, they each discovered the joy of a more similar partner.

Martha recounts that at first their being in love was accompanied by much fear, shame, and modesty, especially from her end. He was unsure whether she really liked him and she was afraid of not being attractive any longer – typical of the somewhat older woman. In her, this uncertainty manifested itself in attacks of extreme timidity, hand in hand with abundant perspiring. He betrayed his sense of insecurity by telling as many witty stories and jokes as possible. But he did something else, too: he praised her by telling her, frequently and aloud, how sweet and attractive he thought she was. Although this was an entirely new experience for Martha, at least in comparison to her marriage, it made her somewhat uncomfortable at first, and her nervousness, in turn, made him uncertain again.

It was an obvious matter of heightened vulnerability for both of them at this stage of life, especially in the sense of: 'Am I still attractive?' This vulnerability is said to be more pronounced in women than in men.[3] It is all the more true when it is a question of romance, when the aging body is once again the centre of attention – if not in reality, certainly in fantasy.

Besides, Martha noted a remarkable change in herself. Where in earlier days she put up with the attentions of gentlemen – to the point where she let herself be loved more than she would choose a partner on her own initiative – this time around she had made her own choice. This was a new experience for her. She had, of course, been in love before, but always on one condition: the other had to have selected her first. Apparently, her narcissism had to be gratified first before she 'was able to see something in him'. This could easily lead to a 'wrong choice'.

Martha sees the turn-around, that of making her choice herself, as obvious progress. Looking back on her life, she has the feeling that this is her first true experience of being in love with a man. She and her partner are available to one another and to their work. They are no longer distracted by urgent obligations towards a third party who depends on them. Their mutual availability offers prospects to the relationship and creates a world of experience that so far has been unknown to Martha.

In Martha and in women like her there is the additional feeling of regret over the loss of the shared life with the previous partner. Moreover, there is a clear sense of the finiteness of existence, the fear of growing old or falling ill, and the sense of haste that may be the result of all of this. Enjoying the present day goes hand in hand with the question: Will we still have time to realize the mutual experiences we have missed and put together a supply of shared experiences? Letting go of the past and of the previous partner continues to be an obvious concern for both of them. It is more difficult to dispose of the feelings and habits one has as one grows older. The most essential stages of life have been lived (with other people), so that there is relatively little common history to fall back on.

Not only did Martha have less positive experiences with her previous partner, she had always had a triple task as woman, wife, and mother as well, with regard to career, husband, and children. That responsibility had weighed heavily on her. In retrospect, it seems to her that this combination had certainly harmed her conjugal relationship. In contrast, Martha experiences her current life as a surprising phase. She had never expected that so many new experiences and even unknown satisfactions would still be open to her.

It was precisely the pressure to live according to stereotypical role patterns that had made her feel so restricted. As these diminished, more space was made for different roles, for reflection, and for the enjoyment of life. In particular, for a woman the possibility of functioning in a more male fashion and for a man to be more feminine, as the literature describes,[4] opens opportunities for partners to better understand each other and function less as each other's opposite.

Martha and her daughter

Martha states that she has a good relationship with her daughter, the youngest child. This is all the more remarkable because she had never had that kind of relationship with her own mother. In Martha's eyes this new experience has produced great benefits for her own further development.

Martha and her daughter have a loving, trusting bond, which, she feels, is more intimate than the one with her two sons, although the relationship with them has certainly always been positive. Both sons did well with their separation and growth towards independence. When the time came, Martha was able to loosen the close connection with her daughter relatively well, too, contrary to what might have been expected. When questioned, Martha actually admits to a sense of relief when her daughter left home and moved in with her boyfriend. It was the girl's first attempt at standing on her own two feet, while the mother entered a new phase of life.

Thanks in part to the successful separation from her daughter, the mother was able to build a new life for herself, like the one she had known before she was married.

To her surprise, a bond developed between Martha and her daughter that she had never enjoyed either with her husband or with her mother, although this did not happen until after the daughter's challenging puberty – equally well described in the literature.[5] From what she recounts, I have the strong impression that the unresolved homo-erotic relationship of love-and-disappointment she had experienced with her mother came to some sort of resolution, as it were, because of the developing solid relationship with her daughter. They were able to console each other and, at the same time, there was room for the daughter's sadness and anger at her mother because of the parents' divorce. In addition, Martha was able to prevent herself from over-burdening her daughter with her own problems. After all, her analysis had taught her to seek counsel within herself where her own dilemmas were concerned.

When the daughter finally fell in love, it aroused very few of the usual feelings of rivalry in Martha, nor did the daughter's leaving home elicit any sense of being abandoned in her. On the contrary, she actually enjoyed being alone after her life with a domineering husband who, just like her mother, had given her little space. Now, when the daughter threatened to restrict her newly acquired space and freedom by clinging to her too much or asking for advice too often, Martha would carefully create the necessary distance again.

It is interesting also that Martha has the explicit sense that her daughter and their mutual relationship had a healthy and healing effect on her and helped her to work through her traumatic past. This may well be an example of what Sigmund Freud called '*Nachträglichkeit*' – that is to say, the phenomenon that childhood experiences may change meaning in the light of new experiences in subsequent phases of development, or, to put it in a nutshell: 'the retroactive reorganization of the personal past'. Similarly, the significance of Martha's analysis grew along with her, and in retrospect she understood much more clearly how her experiences were connected.

The explanation for all of this seems to lie, at least in part, in the excellent processing of becoming a mother herself. Martha was able to use this experience as an incentive for her continued maturation and development as a woman, partly also thanks to her analysis and in spite of the negative experiences with her own mother.

Moreover, some authors consider becoming a mother to be the third separation–individuation phase, after early childhood and puberty, in a woman's life. According to this viewpoint, the woman goes through three separation–individuation phases, not two, like the man.[6] In my opinion, the woman needs these three cycles of the separation–individuation process because at every new developmental step she is confronted anew – and therein she differs from the man – with both her identification with her own mother and her attempts to differentiate herself from this mother.

New insights in the middle years

Martha's story links up with current developments in the formation of psychoanalytic theory about the middle years. This period in life can be a new creative time in which there is as yet a chance to resolve old emotional conflicts and in which new sources of inspiration and creativity can be tapped.[7] Martha is a good example of the stabilization of the sense of self-worth and the positive influence on the feeling of self-worth that the middle years may bring.

To amplify the history of psychoanalytic views on the middle-aged woman, some citations follow. In 1933, Freud wrote:

> It is a well-known fact, which has provided humanity with ample material for complaint, that women often undergo a strange change of character after they have abandoned their genital functions. They become quarrelsome, whining and pedantic, petty and stingy; in short, they display typically sadistic and anal-erotic characteristics that they did not have before, at the time of their femininity. Comedy writers and satirists have always directed their invectives at this 'old dragon' who was once a charming girl, a loving woman, and tender mother. We understand that this change of character corresponds to a regression of sexual life to the pre-genital phase of sadism and anal eroticism, in which we discovered the disposition to compulsive neurosis.[8]

And in 1933 he wrote about the same middle age of the woman as opposed to that of the man:

> However, I can't avoid mentioning an impression that keeps coming up in analytic practice. A man of about thirty seems to us to be a youthful, not entirely mature individual, who we expect will make vigorous use of the possibilities for development that analysis offers him. A woman of the same age, on the other hand, often frightens us with her psychological rigidity and inflexibility. Her libido has taken up definitive positions and no longer seems capable of exchanging them for different ones. Means to further development do not present themselves; it is as if all of life has

been completed and will not be influenced any more, as if the laborious development towards femininity has actually exhausted the potential of the person in question.[9]

Obviously, Freud's view of the woman in her middle years was rather bleak, and in the psychoanalytic world this perspective has only gradually made room for a different viewpoint. The Viennese psychoanalyst Helene Deutsch, one of Freud's students, still expressed herself in rather dark terms about the climacterium (menopause). The psychoanalyst Thérèse Benedek, a young Viennese colleague of Deutsch, sounds more optimistic, but with regard to menopause she still speaks of '*Torschlusspanik*' [panic at the closing of a door], nevertheless.[10] These tokens of an explicitly negative opinion of the woman must be understood against the background of the atmosphere that was then prevalent in psychoanalysis – namely, the primacy of the theory of compulsion and the Oedipus complex. To summarize briefly, this 'male' look at female development holds that the man enjoys the appetites of being-man, while the woman bears the burdens of not having a penis. To make matters worse, she then loses her fertility during the menopause. These sombre messages about being-woman did not come from Freud alone but, oddly enough, from women such as Helene Deutsch and Thérèse Benedek as well, who had certainly themselves never been victimized, who were not masochists, and who often had their most creative periods after their fiftieth year.

Modern psychoanalytic theory sees female development in a much more positive light and, in fact, views the middle years as making room for new experiences. Female sexuality turns out to be far from over when fertility comes to an end. Rather, sexuality turns out to be a function that both sexes can maintain throughout life.[11]

Modern psychoanalytic literature describes middle age as a period in life where object relationships are more central than the drives. Children leaving home, reframing the image of old age when one's own parents turn out to be vulnerable and needy, the approach of death, and the growing awareness of one's own mortality, all upset the narcissistic balance and call for re-orientation. Sigmund Freud no longer needed his younger colleague Carl Gustav Jung as friend and supporter. Once he was certain of what he wanted, he distanced himself from Jung. Having reached middle age, he chose his own path entirely by himself, just as Martha did. As mentioned before, the combination of meaningful relationships, talent, and wisdom can produce a special creativity in this later phase of life.[12]

Parenthood, too, plays a significant role as a developmental stage in the middle years. The period after the children have left home is sometimes called the 'post-parental relaxation'[13] period – referring to the more-or-less constant stress for both parents that accompanies the raising of and caring for children. After this 'emergency phase of parenthood' a calmer period usually sets in for them. The often extremely polarized role pattern of the father who provides and the mother who tends can now make room for relaxation and a whole range of new experiences.

Martha is an example of a successful 'third individuation', as middle age is sometimes labelled[14] – an analogy with the two previous separation–individuation phases, namely the 'psychological birth' in the toddler years and the repetition during adolescence.

The effects of Martha's treatment

In order to take a more detailed and critical look at Martha's line of development, we shall first attempt to draw up a balance sheet of her psychoanalytic treatment, whereby both the positive and the negative aspects must be taken into consideration. In what ways can we see her analysis as successful? And in what aspects can we assume that a better result might have been reached?

A predisposition to gain by treatment always plays an important role, too, of course. In what respects did Martha's re-orientation lead to personal growth, and in what ways did her life stagnate?

We shall begin by scrutinizing the negative aspects in Martha's development. Early in the case description we noted that Martha's fear of her irascible, moody husband resembled in many ways her withdrawal from her capricious and short-tempered mother. Martha's marriage showed characteristics of what Sigmund Freud had already indicated: that the man tends to be the heir of the unresolved relationship with the mother.[15] According to Freud, it is with her (first) husband that a woman tends to thrash out the unresolved intra-psychological conflicts from the early childhood relationship with her mother. Over and over again it can be seen how powerfully the repetition compulsion can make itself known.

This is certainly true in Martha's case. Looking back, she herself sees that in her own experience her first husband was clearly the successor of the mother. Both were sensed as being coercive and restrictive in a traumatic way. For women, a divorce can often be an attempt to free themselves after the fact from the so-called internalized mother. Apparently, in Martha's analysis the relationship with this intra-psychological mother had not been resolved sufficiently to make an unburdened partnership choice possible.

It is likely that, to a great extent, Martha successfully managed to circumvent the negative mother transference, the hate towards the mother that comes back to the analyst. In treatment it is often difficult to make the anger come to the surface. Subsequently, she transferred her angry self to her partner by means of projective identification – that is to say, she projected her own unwanted characteristics onto her husband, so she could thus fight them in him and ensure that they would remain unconscious to herself. He impersonated what and who she did not want to be.

Martha's reservations and fears with regard to the analyst seem to have been worked out insufficiently in the transference. Had this been more successful, probably more 'psychological space' would have been created to help her to 'grasp' and tolerate the anger at the mother (note that this is the infantilized and internalized mother image).

In this context the British psychoanalyst Wilfred R. Bion speaks of 'containing',[16] whereby he refers to the possibility of psychologically working out fantasies that belong to highly primary sensations and reactions, as stimulated by the mother in the earliest years of life. For instance, by articulating the feeling of fear, she helps the child to localize the source of that fear, so that the child's perception of fear can be 'grasped' by him. Similarly, psychoanalytic treatment also aims at changing feelings that cannot be 'grasped' into more manageable thoughts and then furnishing these with a context by fitting them into the life story of the analysand.

Apparently, during treatment Martha had not felt safe enough – an all too common occurrence, unfortunately – to live and expose her fantasy in all its vehemence. She continued to struggle with unconscious, controlled anger, which she projected in part onto her first husband. He impersonated the unconscious, repressed sides of her personality, as it were, for a daughter will do anything to avoid resembling her mother. This is especially true for those of the mother's characteristics of which she disapproves because they had been so burdensome to herself. However, frequently a child involuntarily adopts the very characteristics of a parent that have made it suffer in the past in order to fight that parent with his or her own weapons. Martha had – unconsciously – projected her 'swallowed' mother, who still irritated her, onto her husband and suffered from his disagreeable behaviour in the same way that she used to suffer from her mother earlier.

In addition, there are several positive points to be mentioned. In the first place, it is remarkable that Martha did not repeat the emotional neglect she endured, first from her mother and then from her husband, in the active role with regard to her daughter. For all intents and purposes, the latter was spared the emotional problems of her mother's past. Better yet, Martha was actually able to profit from her daughter's positive development.

With severe problems in the mother–daughter relationship it is consistently noteworthy that the mother clings to the attachment with the daughter in order to silence her own narcissistic issues. Unrequited wishes for love in the marriage, which find their origin in ungratified longings vis-à-vis the mother, often seek gratification from the next generation this way. It is an example of what is sometimes called 'transgenerational transmission, namely the transfer of unresolved emotional problems (such as 'mourning') from one generation to the next. Psychotherapy and/or analysis aim at preventing the repetition of infantile conflicts, and not only with respect to what Sigmund Freud already indicated as '*Wiederholungszwang*', the compulsion to repeat, in the life of the analysand him or herself. It will also prevent the inadvertent transmission of traumatic experiences to the next generation(s).

With Martha, the relationship with her daughter remained unencumbered, despite the fact that in treatment she had only partially resolved the negative mother transference to the female analyst. Apparently, on that point the analysis did have a preventive effect with regard to the daughter. Transgenerational repetition was avoided and even made it possible that a traumatic and frustrating relationship could be replaced by a loving relationship, conducive to growth. In this case, it was obvious that not only can the mother influence the daughter, but the reverse is true as well. In this case the chance for the daughter to have a beneficial influence on the mother's development was substantially increased by the (preceding) psychoanalytic treatment of the mother. It made her open to the restorative effect that a new mother–daughter generation can exert.

A second positive point lies in Martha's experience that in her middle years she landed in a whole new stage of life with very different and as yet unfamiliar possibilities. Martha found a new and more suitable partner and, for the first time in her life, had a relationship with a man that was completely positive and lacked any ambivalence. Her treatment was still sorting out the effect on her experiences, adaptations, and developments in subsequent phases of life. Treatment reverberates for years, so that during new phases of life old issues can still be resolved.

The arrival of Martha's new partner occurred soon after her daughter left home. It seems as if the man is taking her place and thus seems to be heir to the solid mother–daughter relationship. The negative relationship with the mother and the previous partner is not repeated with – that is, passed on to – the new love object. At the time of her analysis, the 'repetition compulsion' was only partially resolved, which led, among other things, to the fact that her unsatisfactory marriage failed in the end.

Third, it should be said that, following the divorce, Martha's obvious period of mourning over what she had lost in her life and what she would never attain was positive and encouraged growth. During this process she gradually regained her sense of self-worth and began to love herself again, which then inspired her to desire love again. She began to 'look around', with the described result. After a while she also regained her self-confidence, in part because of the relationship with her new partner and the certainty that she was loved and appreciated: her narcissistic equilibrium was being restored. It also led to her feeling more in control of her own body and being able to enter for the first time into a captivating, flourishing, and tender sexual relationship. On that level, too, she is no longer the passive woman of yore, when the man had to fall in love with her first and take the initiative with every step. According to Martha, all of this has radically changed.

It triggers greater fear and uncertainty than before to throw oneself into the adventure of a new relationship in this new phase of life. So far, little is to be found on this topic in the literature. However, in my opinion, there are also positive changes connected with the insight into the finiteness of life and with the realization that one should make the most of a newly offered chance. As the years roll on, the idealization that is part of being in love becomes more difficult but is in no way impossible. This shows once again that it is not the so-called objective attraction that is at work when one is in love. Old people can easily find each other physically attractive, despite the wrinkles. It is the work of fantasy that makes imagination powerful, as Sigmund Freud and the French novelist Marcel Proust almost simultaneously noted early in the last century.[17]

In the fourth place, long after her analysis Martha turned out to be able to fully use what she had 'learned' there and put it into practice with a 'fresh' love object. According to the English psychoanalyst Pearl King, the middle phase of life is a kind of reversed puberty: to weather this period in a positive way, it is required that childhood, puberty, and adolescence have been worked through.[18] Apparently, that is exactly what happened in Martha's case.

Psychoanalysis then and now

Martha's psychoanalytic treatment during adolescence took place at a time when psychoanalysts, especially in the Netherlands, were not yet trained very well in handling and processing the fine points of transference and countertransference. Neither were people trained to observe mother–daughter conflicts microscopically and explore the destructive fantasies that can play a part in them. All pathology was still seen in terms of an oedipal relationship and the frustrated amorousness of the girl for the father.

Furthermore, one was frequently referred to the past for all that is actually part of the present, in the here and now of the analytic transference situation. This often led to a more intellectualizing and rationalizing and generally speaking a more explanatory and even pedagogical approach than to a method that aims at emotional interaction, before anything else. Thereby the unconscious fantasy world, which, after all, forms an entirely individual underground mythology, barely had a chance, or at least insufficiently so.

At that time, 'reconstruction', too, was still the magic word – that is to say, in the analysis the situation of the childhood years had to be reconstructed. This promoted a certain preoccupation with what might really have happened, with the question how traumatically parents might have treated the child. Referring back to the assumed 'reality of the past' in this way could easily harm the work of the transference interaction. It was – and still is – very easy to overlook all kinds of utterances that concern the transference relationship. The concealed feelings and fantasies of the analysand with respect to the analyst often went unnoticed, or else one would purposely let sleeping dogs lie in order to circumvent anger. Of course, it was easier for both parties if everything allegedly took place in the past, externally, instead of in the present of the current transference relationship.

When treating the negative transference, I myself also used to prefer sailing around the analysand's aggressive aspirations and feelings of hate for the analyst at the time. The argument was that the dealing with these would harm the therapeutic relationship or cause the patient too much anxiety. However, the contrary is true, as is made clear every time. Through the transference relationship, old feelings are stirred up, not against the parents this time, but against the analyst. This is extremely useful, and even necessary, because it provides the analyst with the sorely needed opportunity to accept these feelings and then to clarify them, so that insight can ensue. Not discussing the fear and anger thus engendered will obstruct any change. It is not enough for parents to make their appearance on the analytic stage, and it is completely inadequate to refer back to the parents as the 'guilty parties'. Analysands themselves must be willing to change. They are responsible for their own life, and their feelings do not merely refer to a distant past: they are active participants in the present. And the only interpretations of the analyst that truly cut any ice are the transference interpretations of the (relived) feelings in the here and now.

A follow-up inquiry, such as the one described here, helps to ascertain that neither psychoanalysis as a science nor the analyst as individual practitioner have been idle in comparison with thirty years ago.

Reviewing Martha

The question remains: What are the factors that can make progressive development in the middle years possible in Martha and in women like her? What inspired the personal growth in the middle years whereby stagnation and regression were averted?

Important were her introspective ability, her curiosity that kept her looking for new experiences and their applications, and – last but not least – her masochistic attitude, which turned out not to be so deeply grounded that it would stop her from changing. The potential for plumbing the depths of her own feelings and use them to understand her own motivations is a form of self-analysis that is often the permanently beneficial result of a treatment that has proceeded well. Besides, Martha was quite able to experience and work through her 'depressive position'.[19] This means that a person can let go of the childlike idea that he or she is the centre of the world and can accept having two parents who were together well before the child entered the stage. One can become an adult only once this has successfully happened – that is, once the individual in question is capable of acknowledging and tolerating his or her position as the third party in the triad between parents and child. Furthermore, Martha was very young when she had the motivation to be treated, and the desire to change her life was her own. Finally, the factors of talent (a feature not readily explicable and hard to define, it is the gift to be able to profit from treatment) and the course of a life, no matter how unpredictable, also play an important role, of course.

Conclusion

This chapter has described the emotional development of a woman in her middle years, which was then compared to new points of view in current psychoanalytic theory, and then also connected to the psychoanalytic treatment of this particular woman in her twenties.

The process outlined above suggests the possibility that analysis can not only prevent a repetition of mother–daughter problems but, in addition, can create space afterwards – '*nachträglich*' as Freud calls it – for the positive experience of being a daughter. It seems that a mother's intra-psychological repair is possible via the subsequent generation, albeit without (the need for) it impacting on the daughter who makes this new identification possible.

The psychological evolution, emotional maturation, and new forms of creativity, as repeatedly described in the literature, were illustrated here in the concrete case history.

Whether for a woman in the middle years her 'anatomy' will also be her 'destiny' depends on her creative ability to furnish her life with substance and direction. The biological clock ticks more loudly for a woman than for a man. The middle years bring a reduction in biological possibilities with them, a physical decline, and a possible psychological regression. However, the fact that all sorts of physical and emotional obligations cease to exist can also be a relief and provide room for new things, as Freud's wife Martha said with a sigh: 'At this age everything becomes a little less difficult for a woman.'[20]

Competence, expertise, experience, and efficiency are all part of the middle years. Finding a new equilibrium in all kinds of areas of life is a development that goes hand in hand with the aging process. Possibilities for leadership, overview, and influence multiply. The middle years are a period in which the personality's repressed aspects and untapped capacities get another chance to be validated as well.

All these things tend to happen later in women than in men. Although in puberty girls mature sexually earlier than boys, erotic maturity – in the sense of finding pleasure in sexuality – usually arrives later for women than for men. The biological clocks of both genders do not run parallel. It does seem that the harmony between genders may be enhanced at a later age, not only because men tend to grow more sensitive but also because women dare to allow themselves greater expansion. Both genders are now inclined to greater reflection and introspection. They attribute a more important role to their mutual relationships,[21] not least because the children no longer stand in the way of romance and eroticism.

The middle years have become an entirely new field of research for psychoanalysis, just as adolescence gained full recognition before, and 'infant research', with the help of video and computer, entered a theretofore unknown peak period. Development theory is gradually being expanded to reach from the earliest beginnings to old age and the end of life.

Chapter 9

On rejected mothers

The fiercest parent–child conflicts typically develop between mothers and daughters, not between fathers and sons, as the Oedipus myth recounts. This chapter deals with daughters who reject their mothers. I give several examples of rejected mothers who were feeling desperate and sought help. If both parties to the conflict are prepared to cooperate, finding a solution is usually possible.

Violent conflicts can erupt between mother and daughter around the birth of a child (the puerperium). This is worth mentioning because that is exactly the time when a daughter needs her mother the most. It is precisely when she most longs for support that she sometimes obstinately rejects her mother. On the other hand, it is also at this time that a resolution to these conflicts is often easier to find, given that around the time of a birth the psychological sluices are more open, as it were.

Conflicts between mothers and daughters – often a life-and-death battle in fantasy – are of all time. The classic example of a daughter who rejects her mother is that of the mythological Electra, as mentioned earlier. As we saw, in her case the unbridled hatred of daughter Electra for mother Clytemnestra actually led to matricide. For thousands of years this tragic tale has been considered psychologically relevant. In this context, it is remarkable that in every ancient and modern version of Electra the viewpoint is that of the daughter. Similarly, in most psychological discussions about parent–child relationships the argument is made from the position of the child, not of the parent. I would like to shed some light on how the situation can present itself when seen from both sides. To my best knowledge very little if anything has been written about the 'rejected mother', and no research has been done on her as far as I know. Therefore, the experiences as described below are entirely my own.

Divorce difficulties

Although I discuss rejected mothers in particular, first some observations about fathers. It needs to be said that rejected fathers are a far more common phenomenon. It is a fate that can strike fathers during and after a divorce, whether or not through their own doing. Because children generally stay with the mother, her influence is greater, and she may involve the children in a loyalty conflict. She can sabotage visitation rights or even make them wholly impossible – something that occurs on a regular basis. When children are struggling with loyalty conflicts after a divorce, it often works out to the disadvantage of the father rather than of the mother.

If, in the eyes of the child, the father has behaved negatively – as in the case of incest, for instance – it can lead to complete rejection of that parent, for understandable reasons. But in less extreme cases, too, divorced fathers often have very little if any access to their children any more. This is the worst solution, especially when in addition the children are turned against the helplessly watching father. When the conflicts between ex-spouses keep smouldering after a bad divorce, they are often thrashed out over the backs of the children. In the most serious cases there is actually little hope for a better understanding later on, when the children are independent.

The father's position after divorce is in part a social problem. It is connected to the law, which gives the mother the more advantageous position with regard to custody of and access to the children. As a father, one can lose wife, children, and house in one fell swoop and, to top it all off, be obliged to pay alimony. When this happens to a father, he is irate, and rightfully so, but is he capable of looking at his own role in the situation as well?

The rejected fathers whom I have seen in my practice usually came because they were angry and offended about the new impasse, rather than because they were feeling miserable about it. The fathers came primarily to justify themselves and clean the slate, not so much to seek their share in the altercation. This may be a coincidence, just as the fact that they were involved with angry daughters rather than sons may be one as well. In contrast, for rejected mothers a vehement sense of failure and guilt almost always dominates.

Why mothers are rejected

What is the situation for mothers who are rejected by their daughter? I have seen a number of examples of this in my practice. Obviously, those who struggle with this problem and seek help do not represent rejected mothers in general. They are largely the ones who feel absolutely miserable and/or guilty in their present situation. They look for help because they are willing to do anything to try to find a resolution to a conflict that is so painful to them. In the best-case scenario, these mothers are wholly disposed to examining their share in the discord provoked. Both mother and daughter feeling miserable about the estrangement is the best condition for treatment. It can be discussed with both parties, and this can bring them closer to each other. It is a bad omen, of course, when the daughter cannot see the mother's step to the psychotherapist as an attempt towards rapprochement and then refuses to react to her mother's request to come and speak with the therapist just once – although preferably more often.

It happens that children do not want to see their parents any more – daughters their mothers – something that in their mind is justified and understandable to an outsider. In *Los van de wereld* [Detached from the world],[1] Hella de Jonge wrote that she had not wanted to see her mother for a year. She recounts in fairly great detail all the conflicts with her parents – two Jewish war victims who survived the war together as younger people. Without any family, they tried to pick up the thread after the war, and this was only partly successful. Traumas do tend to affect subsequent generations. Hella especially recounts the insuperable chasm she felt between her mother and herself. Only when she is told that her mother is dying does she decide to try reconciliation, but by then her mother is unconscious, and she dies an hour later. In such and similar dreadfully sad cases it becomes all the more clear that more than one generation is needed to either ruin or ameliorate relationships definitively between children and parents. In this case, however, it was not merely a question of the war experiences, which were ghastly enough. Hella's mother herself had been badly short-changed emotionally as the child of a mother who was far too young. She had been raised not by her mother but by her grandmother, and she had felt rejected. Grievances about an encumbered past are readily transferred to the children. Mothers easily transmit their unconscious problems to their daughter. After all, the latter is of the same gender and walks in her mother's footsteps. Hella's mother's problem landed especially in the lap of her eldest daughter, the writer of this autobiography.

Not wishing to see a parent again is a last life-saving device in what is, subjectively considered, an intolerable situation, but nevertheless it is regrettable and often causes illness. For evasion is not a solution. The negative bond is more likely to be reinforced by avoiding one another. One can escape from reality, but it is not possible to disengage the disturbing images. By not seeing each other, reality cannot produce a corrective influence on fantasy. Instead, everything is reinforced and enlarged, whereby the imagination continues to rule and exercises its negative influence inside the head of the people involved. Such an evasion can grow into an obsession that takes up a great deal of attention, leads to a great deal of worry, and costs enormous amounts of energy. Sometimes there is no other way out, for there actually are mothers who harm their children and are unable to feel any guilt or regret about it. A heart-rending example can be found in Irène Némirovski's book *Suite française*.[2] She had been emotionally neglected by her Jewish mother, who was murdered in the Second World War. Her children survived and after the war went knocking on the door of their grandmother, who lived in Nice. She did not answer their call for help; she did not even open the door but told them through the keyhole that they had better find shelter in an orphanage.

Fortunately, such seriously disturbed mothers who reject their children and do not suffer from it are rare and, obviously, are not the ones who seek help in psychotherapy. Apparently, not seeing their children or grandchildren causes them no pain. In such extreme cases it is generally the daughter who seeks help, either because she feels guilty, unhappy, or rejected or because she is too angry to ever forgive her mother and is the first to suffer from her embitterment. Unfortunately, it does happen that mothers reject their children, neglect them, or exploit them. However, it is not these violent and unsolvable situations primarily that I want to discuss here. The far less sombre or hopeless cases, where conflicts arise more out of powerlessness, unconscious repetitions of old patterns, and misunderstanding, occur far more often.

When the mother seeks help

Well-meaning, non-understanding, desperate mothers are the ones who seek help because they cannot extricate themselves on their own. Such a mother was Elaine: a pleasant lady in her early sixties, long divorced, who could not understand why her daughter, without any further explanation, always avoided her. A successful businesswoman, the daughter strongly resembled her businesslike, efficient, but emotionally inaccessible father, so said the mother. Perhaps the daughter had already taken her father's side right after the parents' divorce and thought it justified that he had divorced her mother because the two of them seemed less and less suitable for each other. As I listened to Elaine, I tried to put myself in her daughter's position. I could imagine that she had little patience with her mother, although the latter was incredibly well-intentioned. For in myself I also noticed a slight tendency towards impatience when for the umpteenth time she could not understand what I was saying. I did my utmost to formulate everything as simply and clearly as possible. Nevertheless, I often had to repeat my interventions several times in different terms before she would understand me. And even then, the message was still too difficult for the mother, who would answer something like: 'Let me take that down so I can reread it when I get home.' It sounded as if her daughter was an intelligent and analytically thinking woman, a wholly different person from her mother. Parents and children do not always make a good match, and the apple sometimes really does fall far from the tree.

For several years, Elaine came to see me faithfully once a week and, although I felt for her, there was no easy solution. I tried to soften the pain as much as I could while trying to restructure her less-than-wise approach in a positive direction. When she saw her daughter at Grandma's birthday party, she was able to ruin the relationship with her daughter by a tactless remark, which would then again destroy the atmosphere for some time to come. Her daughter had no regular partner and, from what Elaine said, did not seem to be a particularly happy woman. I tried to cultivate better understanding for her daughter in Elaine in order to build a bridge between them that way, but nothing worked.

Whenever possible, I try to work with both mother and daughter. However, in Elaine's case I did not succeed in getting both parties to see me. The daughter refused to come; she went off to live abroad and continued to avoid her mother. One of the rare times they would see each other, though they would hardly speak, was at the annual golf competitions, in the presence of other players, or at a crowded family reunion where there was no opportunity either for any personal contact.

Madame de Sévigné and George Sand: Two scorned mothers

As mentioned earlier, the mother–daughter problem is as old as the hills. Take the famous seventeenth-century epistolary writer Madame de Sévigné. This Parisian lady, who frequented the highest circles of the court, tried in her letters to express her love for her daughter, who had gone to live in the south of France, but it was all in vain. Her letters sound more like passionate declarations of love than like the correspondence between a mother and daughter. The latter stubbornly continued to avoid her mother. She did send her little daughter to spend time with the grandmother, but only because she herself had no interest in raising the child. Contemporaries who witnessed all of this called the daughter '*une vraie Cartésienne*', which essentially means that she was a dry, businesslike soul (in reference to the French philosopher René Descartes, who said 'cogito ergo sum', meaning 'I think therefore I am').

George Sand, a popular nineteenth-century novelist, was also rejected by her daughter, a fact from which she suffered a great deal. Although she lived apart from her husband and occasionally changed lovers, she was a good mother.

In such cases of well-meaning mothers and 'unruly' daughters it seems to be a matter of mutual incomprehension and incompatible characters – a case of a child not being able to recognize him- or herself in a parent or in both parents, resulting in mutual lack of understanding and distancing.

Rejection around a postnatal depression

Denise was a complicated case of a rejected mother. The question here had to do primarily with an unstable daughter who made unsuccessful attempts at keeping her strong mother figure at a distance. On the other hand, the mother, a solid social worker who had lost her own mother when she was quite young, wanted at all costs to be present at the birth of her grandchild. The daughter, who actually wanted to be freed from her mother, would rather not have her there. However, she did not feel she was up to the task of giving her this message herself: her husband, who himself had a bone to pick with his own strongly domineering mother, was to convey the message. He was happy to do so, for it gave him the opportunity to project his anger at his mother onto his mother-in-law.

When she came to me, Denise was on the verge of despair. Her story gave me the impression that the daughter did not feel she could cope with her well-intentioned mother who gave a lot of unsolicited advice. The conflict between son-in-law and daughter had got completely out of hand. Mother-in-law and son-in-law had literally attacked each other physically, while he had added verbal abuse, flinging the most offensive possible words at her.

Upon hearing the mother's account, and having done my utmost to put myself in the place of each of the people involved in the conflict, I did also want to hear the daughter's story. She was willing to come, and what I saw was a sad and vulnerable young woman in a slightly confused state. She began to weep almost immediately when she started to tell her side of the story. It soon became clear to me that the young mother was suffering from postnatal depression, which threatened to victimize three generations. She was deeply sad about the situation and felt more guilt than anger. She had not meant it that way at all, she had not wanted to exclude her mother. On the other hand, she also wanted to try to prevent her mother's far too forceful meddling in her and her family's life. After this conversation, I saw mother and daughter together a few times, at which time I attempted to clarify each of their respective positions to the other. Such arguments are usually founded on misunderstandings and prejudices, especially people who live in close proximity to each other assume they know what the other is thinking without asking for confirmation.

With Denise, unconscious motives played the main role, and this robbed her of her view of reality. Her past caused her to be overly involved as a grandmother with the birth of her grandchild. As a toddler, Denise had lost her mother, who died in childbirth with her second child. This made her more than usually anxious about everything that can go wrong at the time of a delivery. This is understandable: birth lies on the borderline between life and death and always unleashes many emotions. In the period around childbirth the feelings of the young mother come closer to the surface, and a therapist often has easier access. As said, the sluices are open, literally and figuratively speaking. I had already done all the preparatory work with Denise and, after a few conversations with the two of them together, the air was cleared to such an extent that the sharp edges were gone. Both parties were willing to look for solutions. Moreover, it was noteworthy and no accident that Denise's husband was barely involved in the matter. A father who is aloof and lets mother and daughter struggle alone with their conflicts, is incapable of or unwilling to intervene as a facilitator. Such a father neglects his role as arbiter when mother and daughter are too ferocious in their interaction. He should be the one who can facilitate the necessary separation. Fortunately, reconciliation was reached through the discussions, and mother and daughter spontaneously came to new agreements on how to continue their relationship in the future. To everyone's gratification, when the second baby arrived a year later, the problem was not repeated.

A psychoanalytic mother–daughter pair at war

The history of psychoanalysis has also produced a striking example of mother hatred. As a psychoanalyst, Melanie Klein was one of Sigmund Freud's younger contemporaries, though in no way a blind follower of his. On the contrary, she had her own ideas about the development of the child and further expanded Freud's theory by involving particularly the mother in the story. Her vision went back to birth and the earliest phases of development. Klein assumed that there exists a father–mother–child triad from the very onset. Not only the mother, but the father, too, is present from the beginning. He does not just appear at the end of the fifth year of life, when for Freud the oedipal stage appears. Furthermore, she was also convinced of the importance of the transference relationship in children. The feelings towards those who raise the child are most definitely transferred onto the therapist.

In the 1920s Klein moved from Vienna to London at the invitation of her colleague Ernest Jones. There she continued to elaborate and disseminate her theories on child development, to the great displeasure of Freud's daughter, Anna, who, after fleeing from the Nazis with her father and mother in 1938, had also settled in London as a children's psychoanalyst. Throughout her life she would continue to hold fast to her father's vision and protect his legacy by fire and sword. The controversy grew to be so intense that, as a result of the drama between the two ladies, two separate psychoanalytic directions were created in the British Psycho-Analytical Society. Heated discussions in that Society took place during the Second World War.[3] Under the bombers' loud roar, Anna Freud (whose father had died in the interim) and Melanie Klein thrashed out their theoretical war. The conflict in and of itself began to closely resemble a mother–daughter battle, for Melanie was considerably older than Anna. Furthermore, the two ladies had sufficient cause for a life-and-death battle: each of them hated her own mother. However, this turned out to be only the prelude to the murderous mother–daughter feud that was to follow.

The latter was sparked when Klein's daughter, Melitta Schmideberg, involved herself in the struggle. She is a fine example of a daughter who initially follows enthusiastically in her mother's footsteps. Emulating her, she became a psychoanalyst as well. She then had a conflict with her mother and thus landed in the other camp. Gradually, her hate for her mother increased progressively, to the point that she actually emigrated to America.

This particular mother–daughter conflict became more widely known in general thanks to the play by Nicholas Wright, *Mrs. Klein*.[4] The ferocity of this play, a variant on the Electra theme, defies all description. Melanie Klein can be blamed for taking on her own children into analysis and using them to support her psychoanalytic ideas. Obviously, something like this is entirely at odds with a mother's role and seriously damaging to the emotional bond with her children. Such practices laid the foundation for the subsequent fierce hatred of her daughter Melitta who, without any qualms, rejected her mother vehemently and publicly.

The most aggressive collisions between mothers and daughters run across several generations. The bad relationship with one's own mother is projected onto the daughter later on. Klein's daughter became the victim of the fact that Klein herself had loathed her own mother.

Emotionally vulnerable mothers

If matters can disintegrate so badly between ordinary mothers and daughters, one can imagine how hard it must be for psychologically disturbed mothers to have a good relationship with their daughters. There are mothers who are so unstable that they are kept at a safe distance because they are too hard to handle. Such a one is Sandra, a mother who holds extreme views on food. She claims that eating anything other than raw food and drinking pure fruit juices is not only unhealthy but actually life-threatening; and she does not keep this bizarre conviction to herself but spreads it as if she is part of a proselytizing mission. Her conviction has all the characteristics of religious mania, except that it concerns food, not God. When the daughter who is just feeding her first baby has had enough, she firmly throws her mother out. In the overly sensitive period after childbirth something like this leads to a confrontation more swiftly.

The association with a disturbed mother requires an adjusted approach that can be learned, with some help. The daughter must learn to accept that her mother has not given her what she could normally have expected from her. This is followed by a lengthy mourning process and renunciation of the hope that what was longed for might still come. The daughter begins to see that her mother has serious shortcomings and is emotionally disturbed. Such a daughter will reflect upon the association with her mother and try to get the initiative on her side. She will set her limits more clearly: 'this far and no further'. Thus she creates the conditions that will enable her to make fewer concessions as regards the length and frequency of the contact between them.

Sandra is the typical demanding, coercive mother. Insecure mothers who are afraid that their children do not love them have a tendency to kindle guilt feelings in them. That way they try to force them to pay the attention they fear they are losing. Such a mother will try to impose her will and her opinion, come high or come low. As stated before, it often concerns insecure mothers who toss their defencelessness and helplessness into the ring as their weapon. Or else it concerns psychologically disturbed mothers who project their fears onto their child. Drawing the line will then be absolutely mandatory. One should not make a vulnerable, self-doubting mother anxious or insecure by beginning a battle with her, as Melitta Schmideberg, Melanie Klein's daughter, did. Predictability is important. Clear-cut agreements about regularity and continuity provide security and prevent fear in the mother. Mother and daughter both know where they stand. The daughter guards her perimeters and is consistent in the agreements made. Even when no deals can be made, an implicit regularity that the daughter sets up with herself can work well. That way a mother who feels easily rejected will not become unnecessarily rattled, and the contact will get out of hand less quickly.

Attraction and repulsion

Sometimes daughters claim they do not want to see their mother any more because she is always brimming over with unwanted advice for them. However, this often turns out to be a fire that both parties ignite. It seems as if the daughter still finds herself in puberty. She still knocks on her mother's door with her worries and problems, and then, when the latter interferes, the daughter becomes irate. To her great exasperation she is treated like a child again. This eliciting and rejecting of any help and advice is based on the daughter's puberty-like protest that ought to become conscious if she wants to break down the pattern. Puberty is an important developmental phase in which the ability to react and protest against the parents is of overriding importance. The phase offers indispensable opportunities for the acquisition of independence. When these are not used and there has been no question of any resistance or protest, it will be less favourable for a child's aggression management. It is not hard for the therapist to discern that an adult woman has skipped something essential in her development, whereby handling and regulating anger has been insufficiently practised or has sometimes actually failed completely. This omission interferes with the emergence of her own interests and the establishment of clear-cut perimeters. I knew an adult woman whose mother committed suicide after the first confrontation with her daughter's anger. Thereby she still succeeded in causing her daughter lifelong guilt feelings from the grave.

When a mother abandons her family

A different category of rejected mothers are those who abandon their families prematurely, sometimes when the children are still quite young. In that case, the father is left behind with the child or children, and often fairly quickly finds a replacement partner who will take on the arduous role of stepmother and wife. The end of the story is that the actual mother no longer has access to her family or her children. Tolstoy's riveting tale of Anna Karenina is a classic example of this. She falls in love with a young officer, which causes such a scandal that her much older husband denies her any access to their child, so that she can no longer see her little son. One night she sneaks into the conjugal home to embrace her child one last time. Not long thereafter the officer's love begins to wane, and Anna feels so desperately lost and lonely that she decides to throw herself under a train: there is, after all, no way back for her any more.

Children who are abandoned by their mothers end up in such a fierce loyalty conflict that usually they can do nothing but, in their turn and under the pressure of the new set of parents, reject the 'aberrant mother'.

Moyra was already in her early fifties when she came to me for the first time. She had last seen her daughter, born from a mixed marriage, when the girl was 4 years old. After the child was born, the husband, a foreign-born Muslim, had suddenly set traditional demands for his Dutch wife. Henceforth she was to stay at home, not work any more, and lead the life of a Muslim woman geared exclusively to her own and her extended family. All of this came as a total surprise to Moyra. She had not expected it from her highly educated husband. When she would not submit, he threatened to kill her. Moyra fled her home and later divorced him. This drama had taken place some 25 years before, but Moyra, who had remarried, still could have no peace with the thought that she did not know her child. What she found especially and increasingly more painful was the question from total strangers whether she had any children. She simply could not decide whether she should answer that query positively or negatively, and in social situations she felt increasingly helpless and uncertain. At her wits' end, she wanted to hire a detective and have him find out where her daughter might be, so she could try to take up contact again. It did not seem a wise plan to me, and I counselled her that we first spend some time together to discuss all the implications of such a step.

We began a therapeutic process that provided her with greater insight into her motives. She was not in the least aware of her shame and her feelings of guilt. First and foremost, it seemed necessary to me that she become conscious of her fears and fantasies. After we had been involved with this for more than a year, a member of her ex-husband's family happened to telephone her and could tell her where the lost daughter lived. Apparently, she had married in the meantime and now had a family of her own. Moyra was elated and wanted to pursue this immediately. After we had discussed all the risks involved, she decided to attempt a first contact by letter, expecting that she would soon be welcomed with open arms. Unfortunately, such was not the case. It took a great deal of trouble to make her understand that patience was more appropriate here than speed. After all these years, a period of mutual exploration would be needed. Greater insight and Moyra's will-ingness to acknowledge her daughter's indignation would be a condition for a successful first encounter. Moyra found it far too patently obvious that her child would be thrilled to have her mother back, although that was not very plausible. It would be hard to believe that the daughter would have felt any-thing but betrayed by her mother. Furthermore, the daughter's loyalty was for her stepmother and her father, not for her mother. She had been told that her own mother had died and fully considered her stepmother as her own mother. By renewing contact with her mother after all these years, she would certainly bring down upon herself her father's and stepmother's hatred. The daughter was not prepared to relinquish her loyalties for someone unknown.

Moyra had to learn to understand that a child does not simply continue to love a prematurely vanished mother. Initially she wanted nothing to do with the anger that her daughter must undoubtedly have felt for her. It seemed to me that without acknowledging this absolutely legitimate anger, there could be no question of any reconciliation. Moyra had a difficult time recognizing, not to mention accepting, that the abandoned child's reproach and anger were inevitable. She had, after all, acted out of pure despair. To me Moyra kept insisting that she was overflowing with positive maternal feelings and itching to show her love. She wanted to hear nothing of the inevitable guilt feelings about her original handling of things, which she had completely repressed. The confrontation with her fierce denial caused her to become furious with me for the first time. Moyra's outburst let me know that we were on the right track. A mother who abandons her child cannot help but be prey to shame and feelings of guilt, no matter how understandable or legitimate her motives may have been. Her unconscious guilt feelings made her blind to the fact that her daughter might be vindictive towards her. The key word for both parties in this case was forgiveness. When a mother can forgive herself for her mistakes, she will no longer need to deny them or to feel excessively guilty. But the child, too – the daughter, in this case – can only let go of her anger about grief suffered when she is able to forgive her parents for their shortcomings. Parents are not as omnipotent as they seem to a child. Later on, the insight grows that parents, too, had parents and circumstances that were decisive in their lives. They do not always act out of conscious motives, but more often out of powerlessness, ignorance, or the projection of unconscious motivations. A parent can see an enemy in a child, for example, when she projects onto her child her own parent, with whom things did not mesh. Or she may see her husband from whom she is divorced in her son or daughter: 'You are just like your father.'

Moyra had the fantasy that she would be warmly welcomed, as is often seen in TV series or soap operas about reunions, but, of course, in real life things are never that simple, and disappointment always lurks. When after many long years a child meets a lost parent, the problems are only just beginning, for everything is not immediately forgiven and forgotten at the allegedly happy reunion of two almost complete strangers.

I had a different but similar case with a somewhat happier ending, although the road that led there was laborious and long as well. It concerned Maria, a mother who could not possibly endure sticking it out with her husband. She fled her home, leaving her two young children behind. The husband remarried, and Maria herself found a new marriage partner as well.

After her ex-husband died, she tried to make contact with his widow in an attempt to gain access to her children again. It turned out that she was not welcome; she then sought therapeutic help to figure out how to handle the situation. Her children did not immediately react to her efforts, which ended up as a process of finding favour, providing financial assistance, and demonstrating her good intentions that went on for years, with her current husband's support. Slowly the bonds were strengthened and some contact was re-established, which increased as the children became less dependent on their stepmother.

Further information and patterns

The mother–daughter relationship is a source of ambivalence even under normal circumstances. Every girl has mixed feelings around the strong bond with and the great dependency on her mother. A mother is both her daughter's prop and stay, but also the one who stands in the way of the girl's independence, with all the reproaches and rancour this entails. Boys do not need to follow in their mother's footsteps, they do not go through the same life cycle, and from the very start they are given greater freedom by their mothers and are left more to their own devices.

A girl emulates her mother, and it is from her that she learns mothering so that the generations can succeed each other harmoniously. However, when this fails, it may take several generations before the damage is repaired. In the case of a deceased mother, a psychotic mother, a neglectful mother, or one who leans too heavily on her children, the emotional connections are disrupted.

Mother–daughter relationships often encompass two extremes and all the gradations between these. On the one hand we see mothers who keep their daughters so closely attached to them that we can speak of a symbiotic illusion, which amounts to an idyll that is supposed to camouflage the discord. In such cases the interaction between mother and daughter is especially intense, as if they cannot do without each other. They chat, they telephone each other all the time, but, upon inquiry, there is no question of any true intimacy at all. The mother merely assumes that her child agrees with her, feels the same way she does, has no desire for any distance, and wants nothing more than to have a bond with her. When mother and daughter are in league against the father, the difference between the generations is lost, with all the disturbing consequences this entails. The triangular father–mother–child relationship has become a dyad, a dialogue, from which it is hard to escape. In such a conniving, oppressive relationship there is no room for any difference, especially not for any difference of opinion. Everything goes as if there is no question of any anger, even though – consciously or not – the daughter will feel trapped. She rightfully assumes that her rather unassertive mother is unable to withstand any criticism or protest. She adjusts to the attitude that she senses her mother expects of her and that will be most profitable to her, and thereby she trades independence for love and security.

The other extreme is a mother who is absent, detached, or uninterested and does not aspire to or is incapable of any intimacy with her daughter. In that case an uncompleted longing is created in the daughter who continues to strive for moments of closeness, accord, and recognition. If all of that is doomed to failure and there is no hope for any gratification of fundamental needs for love, it will – whether consciously or unconsciously, openly expressed or not – become a seedbed for fierce animosity against the mother figure.

These are the two extremes between which the normal happy medium of a healthy relationship between mother and daughter can be found. The margin is quite wide, for children are flexible on the whole so that recovery remains possible. The attitude of the father plays an important role here. He ought not to leave the mother–daughter duo to fend for themselves too much. He would be wise to intervene every so often, to curb the mother and support the daughter, if need be. In short, the father has an important function in guaranteeing the family equilibrium and safeguarding the triangular relationship. There is a reason why children have two parents who can complement each other and clarify the existence of different viewpoints to a child. The child's mental development requires the insight that different people can have different thoughts.

In the course of their lives, girls have to deal with repeated periods during which they fall back on their mothers. Progress is constantly interrupted by regressive episodes. The girl follows in her mother's footsteps at the time of her first menstruation, her first sexual experience, pregnancy and childbirth, and even at menopause. At every new phase she again identifies with her. She will compare herself and, when possible, will want nothing more than to have her mother's advice and support. Unfortunately, however, this can also lead to fear of fusion, with avoidance as the result. Daughters are frequently flung back and forth between, on the one hand, a generally unconscious longing for fusion with the mother, and, on the other, the fear thereof. Many women are preoccupied with not wanting to resemble their mothers, which is impossible. The longing for fusion that is sensed as dangerous leads to a fear of proximity. This problem of hold-onto-me-let-me-go does not apply to boys but is all the more applicable to girls. The daughter's inner conflicts, of which mothers tend to be unaware, can lead to their being avoided or even totally rejected. Neurotic conflicts lead rather quickly to misunderstandings between two people. They see each other as something about which the other has no clue. Well-intentioned mothers can make desperate and fruitless attempts to win (back) the love of their daughters. Parents have no leg to stand on, and they have much to lose, such as not being permitted to see their grandchildren. This makes them feel more keenly dependent on their children's tokens of love. Perhaps in order to be able to understand these intricacies, it is necessary to grow older oneself. In their powerlessness, parents – mothers in particular

– resort to provoking guilt feelings, for instance by calling and saying: 'So, are you still alive?' or, when a daughter visits, making a reproach such as: 'Do you have to leave already, you just got here!'

All of this shows how problematic it is to create a person in your own image, as a mother does when she gives birth to a daughter. Creation can go wrong, as in Genesis. In the Biblical tale, God becomes enraged with the disobedient human whom he has created in his own image. He drives Adam and Eve out of Paradise like naughty children, and the first symbiosis is brutally disrupted. He then destroys his own creation by unleashing a Flood on man and animal, and, finally, as punishment for insubordination, he reduces Sodom to ashes. In precisely the same way, the mirror between mothers and daughters can have consequences that are not always entirely good, but can also be the cause of mutual hate and destruction.

Chapter 10

History and hysteria

It is time to place the mother–daughter story in its historical perspective. This chapter deals with the history and the various backgrounds of psychoanalytic theory as they relate to female development. Well over a hundred years ago, in 1895, *Studien über Hysterie* [Studies on Hysteria] by Josef Breuer and Sigmund Freud appeared, marking the beginning of a new century in psychiatry.[1] This work was based entirely on experiences with female patients and should certainly be incorporated here, even though the mother–daughter relationship was in no way part of it yet.

Psychoanalysis was born at the end of the nineteenth and the beginning of the twentieth century out of listening to and treating women. Hysteria – for that was what those women suffered from – once served as the model for the theory on neurosis. Although hysteria thus prevailed as a prototype – for repression and other neurotic mechanisms – this particular diagnosis has all but disappeared today. It has been deleted from the diagnostic manuals of psychiatry, where in just a few words every syndrome is described.[2] The concept of hysteria encompasses too many symptoms that threaten to make it too vague. Nevertheless, the question continues to arise whether hysteria, still somewhat commonly used in psychoanalysis, actually exists or not. A historic overview of the developments over the past hundred years may help to evaluate the usefulness of the concept of hysteria.

For a long time the father–daughter relationship was considered central. We have seen this in Sigmund Freud's case description of Dora, to which he gave the subtitle 'Fragment of an analysis of a case of hysteria'.[3] According to him, the Oedipus complex, the little girl's love for the father in this case, was at the core of every neurosis. I have argued that for girls the relationship with the mother is more central. Additionally, I have argued that the female Oedipus complex is not the same as that of the male and that a different model presents more of a solution. This is the model that I have named the Electra complex, not as a replacement of the Oedipus complex but as a complement thereto. Not every woman has an Electra complex, but the designation is valid when complications in the mother–daughter relationship impede normal development.

History

For a long time hysteria was seen as an emotional disturbance in women, caused by a 'floating' uterus. Inspired by the Greek word for uterus – *hysteros* – emotionally disturbed women were already known as hysterical in the days of antiquity, but it was not until the end of the eighteenth century that hysteria not only became linked with the nervous system instead of the uterus, but was also considered to be a mental disorder.[4] This development opened the way to the scientific study of hysteria, which became the primary focus, for the first time on a grand scale, for the Parisian psychiatrist Jean Martin Charcot at the end of the nineteenth century. Freud studied with Charcot for eight months. A few years later, the authors of the *Studies on Hysteria* broke with the tradition of neurology and tried to provide a psychological explanation for hysteria. Even at that time Sigmund Freud already found it a difficult diagnosis to delineate: 'It is not an independent clinical entity', he wrote.[5]

Currently, hysteria is often subdivided into 'histrionic', 'borderline', and 'narcissistic' personality disorders with hysterical features.[6] Just as Freud thought a hundred years ago, the general opinion today is that hysterical characteristics can appear in different syndromes. Also, the various character-istics of the histrionic personality have been more extensively described.[7]

Freud's teacher Charcot did take psychological factors into account up to a point, but he was still primarily interested in physical causes.[8] Despite his polemical tone towards the well-known nineteenth-century French psych-iatrist Pierre Janet, Freud actually demonstrates a closer kinship to the latter than to Charcot.[9] Although Freud still had to free himself from his predeces-sors and mentors, *Studies on Hysteria* can be seen as the starting point of psychoanalysis, which Freud will mention by that name for the first time in the year 1896.[10]

The most important conclusion of the *Studies* is that emotionally loaded and insufficiently expressed experiences will cause disorders. They will then be repressed and remain active in a split-off part of the psyche that is inaccess-ible to consciousness. '*Der Hysterische leide grösstentheils an Reminiscenzen*' [Hysterics suffer mainly from reminiscences]. The traumatic memories vanish, but anything reminiscent of those memories is painful and leads to avoidance in any way possible. A psychological trauma, consisting of unpleasant mem-ories and reprehensible thoughts that have to be repressed, becomes the basis of an emotional disorder expressed in symptoms.

However, the question remained why an experience, split off from con-sciousness, would remain active in the unconscious. In order to explain this mysterious phenomenon, Freud's co-author Breuer came up with the term 'hypnoid'. He used it to refer to a dissociative, altered state of consciousness, leading to strange behaviour, by which the patient expresses the fact that something is preying on his or her mind. The patient would develop symp-toms like paralysis or sleepwalking, or be unable to speak or to walk. These complaints could be resolved by questioning patients under hypnosis about their condition and what they remembered about its cause – namely, the trauma. The memories that would surface as a result were examined one by one for their reference to the trauma, and this eventually helped the symptoms to disappear.

The importance of *Studies on Hysteria* for psychoanysis

Sigmund Freud's thinking about hysteria resulted in the formulation of his theory of the unconscious. Therein lies the most important philosophical revolution that the *Studies* brought about. Undesirable contents were stored separately from consciousness by means of dissociation and splitting. They were not gone, they were repressed.

Although it had a somewhat different meaning, in Freud's time the unconscious was not unknown as a concept. The field of force in the psyche between various incompatible motives was also known. Janet used this to explain how socially undesirable or forbidden thoughts, such as sexual fantasies, were kept outside consciousness.[11] Freud's dynamic unconscious, drives that forcefully aspire to being expressed, was as new as his idea to involve the relationship between patient and therapist in the treatment.

Freud and his co-author Breuer designated the unconscious as 'split-off', 'dissociated' from consciousness (not yet as repressed). 'Splitting' leading to dissociative disorders – altered states of consciousness, multiple personalities – a term coined by Janet, is currently in use again. Modelled on Melanie Klein's frequent use of the term, splitting has always been central among the Kleinians. She spoke of the 'good' and the 'bad' mother, the two sides of one individual divided among two persons, mother and witch, as in the fairy tales. Another case of splitting is that of a mother who divides her ambivalent feelings between two children, one of whom appears to her as ideal and the other as insufferable. Similarly, dividing experiences between the conscious and the unconscious part of the psyche is also a case of splitting. In the 1970s the US psychoanalyst Otto Kernberg adopted this concept and used it to explain what he calls the 'hysterical personality'. It is remarkable how well the viewpoint of the *Studies* connects both with modern cognitive psychology and with contemporary psychoanalysis.

With the publication of the *Studies*, a revolution took place, not only in the theoretical area but also in the therapeutic one. Both Freud and Breuer would listen daily for hours on end to their patients' highly detailed complaints. At that time, these were primarily women who were regarded more as underage children than as adults by their male contemporaries – witness the plays by the Viennese Arthur Schnitzler and the Swedish Henrik Ibsen, among others.[12] As they listened, these pioneers abandoned the field of neuro-psychiatry to seek psychological patterns that might explain the often bizarre symptoms. Unalterable and indemonstrable 'facts' such as heredity, degeneration (in the sense of being inferior in body and/or mind), and constitution were pushed to the back as much as possible in favour of more psychological explanations.

Initially, Breuer and Freud used catharsis (a Greek word for purification and reconciliation) to make hysterical symptoms disappear. They treated mainly conversions – emotions expressed in body language and as all sorts of physical symptoms. Their method consisted of letting the patients verbalize their old emotions and in so doing bring them to life again. In *Studies on Hysteria* psychosexual development, which later became the leading principle for Freud, was not yet prominent as an explanation for the origin of hysteria. The two men examined every complaint in the smallest detail in order to make connections with traumatic experiences as a possible cause. This endeavour was not merely time-consuming, it was also far from satisfactory. Breuer had developed the method with his brilliant patient Bertha Pappenheim, alias Anna O, the later feminist and social innovator. She came up with her own 'talking cure' and 'private theatre' (her inner world where everything was played out) and referred to her cure as 'chimney-sweeping'.[13]

The concept of hypnoid, newly invented by Breuer, was abandoned in Freud's contribution to the *Studies*, for he did not believe in it. The two authors of the *Studies* did not always see eye to eye. In its final chapter, written by Freud and dealing with psychotherapy, he concludes caustically that the concept of hypnoid explains nothing. According to him, the cause behind the complaints is, upon further reflection, always sexuality.[14] Freud also lost his confidence in the healing power of catharsis. He called it combating symptoms, which helps only when spontaneous recuperation had also set in. With barely concealed scorn Freud concluded that Breuer was doing Sisyphus work with Anna O. Indeed, shortly after the publication of the *Studies*, the two men came into serious conflict. Freud blamed his former mentor for denying the importance of sexuality and in the end wanted nothing more to do with him.

After discarding techniques such as hypnosis, '*Kopfdruck*' (head-pressing: Freud had the habit of putting pressure on his patients' head while asking them to free-associate), and massage, Freud was more inclined to be led by the free brainwaves of his patients. He became fascinated by phenomena that he called defence and resistance. This referred to the patient's tendency to deny offensive fantasies and drives, such as sexuality, and to resist the therapist's attempts to bring them to the surface. In the *Studies* problems around '*Gegenwille*' [defence and resistance] and '*Übertragung*' [transference] – including '*Übertragungsliebe*' [transference love], which would not be named until later and refers to the famous as well as notorious amorous transference to the therapist – were brought to the fore for the first time. That psychoanalysis could actually not succeed without working through the mutual therapeutic relationship, the 'transference', Freud would experience painfully enough later on with his patient Dora,[15] as the sad affair around Sabina Spielrein and her Swiss therapist Carl Gustav Jung would also show.[16] This Russian woman had fallen in love with Jung, who began a relationship with her, whereupon he called on Freud for help to protect him from scandal.

In any event, the research into hysteria had led to the development of psychoanalysis: an intensive treatment based on the revolutionary idea that by way of 'free association' unconscious thoughts can be pointed out and revealed. The patient states freely what comes into his or her mind, and an emotional relationship is formed with the therapist. The transference of old feelings to the latter that is thus created will not be satisfied but will be examined for the benefit of new insight.

Not only were the new psychological perceptions of the *Studies* reasonably well received at the turn of nineteenth and into the twentieth centuries, but many ideas in Freud's chapter on the psychotherapy of hysteria, such as the analysis of the transference, defence, and resistance, are considered still valid today.

The concept of trauma

In the early days of psychoanalysis the concept of trauma played a crucial role. It concerns psychological trauma – that is, the impact of a given event on the psyche. The roles of the external and internal world are clearly distinguished in this. The psychological equilibrium is usually not disturbed by the objective event as much as it is by the meaning that the individual confers on it. Freud had already established before 1895 that trauma is linked to the representation of real or imagined experiences. Thus it becomes comprehensible that the fantasy of being raped can work just as traumatically as an actual rape. We now know that trauma mostly consists not of one single event but of a series of persistently damaging situations, such as parents who fight continuously and the child's fears and fantasies that go hand in hand with this.

According to Josef Breuer, traumas appear in different guises: long-term caretaking of a sick father, grief over an unhappy love, the witnessing of an erotic scene. He was less enthusiastic than Sigmund Freud about sexual traumas as the sole explanation for neurosis. Although by the end of the nineteenth century psychiatry fully acknowledged the significance of sexual feelings, the subject did not yet occupy a prominent place in the *Studies* because of Breuer's influence, although the difference of opinion between the two authors is already tangible. It is likely that Breuer curbed Freud in this respect, for both before the *Studies* and right after the rupture between them sexual trauma came to be the central explanation for Freud. He himself said: 'When I began to analyze the second patient, Mrs. Emmy v. N., I didn't yet believe in sexual aetiology at all. I had only recently left the school of Charcot and considered the connection of hysteria with the theme of sexuality as a kind of indignity – precisely as the patients themselves tend to do.'[17]

Freud grew more and more convinced of the sexual origin of neurosis. For a few years he was wholeheartedly preoccupied with the concept of trauma in the sense of sexual seduction. He was inclined to generalize in the hope that he would suddenly become famous and rich – not an unusual or impossible aspiration in that vibrant period full of new discoveries. While talking with patients, he became convinced that the abuse of the child – whether or not by a parent, but as a rule by the father – was the cause of every neurosis. At the same time he realized that he felt attracted to his daughter Mathilde, but that this did not necessarily mean that he might be inclined to incest. Nor did he believe, as an explanation for his own personal neurotic complaints, that his own father could have been capable of something similar.[18] Thus his theory lost its bearings, and he was leaning towards an entirely different explanation.[19]

Around 1897, after the death of his father and a growing depression, Freud started his self-analysis, during which he discovered the oedipal yearnings he had harboured as a child for his beautiful, young mother. The importance of psychic reality, the internal experience, dawned upon him ever more.[20] He discovered that the fantasy around it is more decisive than any concrete event. One's own interpretation of an event is what matters. Within a few years the abandonment of the seduction theory was a fact. In contrast to the claims of fashionable Freud-bashers,[21] this did not come out of the blue and was not inspired by gain or self-interest. Abandoning his fervent conviction was a gradual and painful process for Freud.[22] He decided that blaming the father as seducer was no solution to the enigma. From that moment on, the fantasies, wishes, fears, and yearnings that the child feels with regard to its parents became central. Freud never denied the magnitude of sexual traumas such as incest, but they no longer had the overpowering weight that he had originally attributed to them. As a result of the rejection of the seduction theory, the incidence of incest and violence against children and their traumatic influence have been on the back burner for all too long. Psychoanalysis has been rightfully held responsible for this and has itself reverted as well.

Dora

That his original idea remained important for Sigmund Freud can be seen in the seduction traumas he attributed to his patient Dora. Dora was a recalcitrant adolescent who had become trapped in her milieu and, unfortunately, received little compassion from 'father' Freud. Besides, in my opinion, the theory around the Oedipus complex is, in Dora's case description, less founded than has always been, and still is, assumed. In psychoanalysis, hysteria and the Oedipus complex were for a long time more or less synonymous, so that Dora's frustrated love for her father simply had to be the cause of her neurosis. Freud and his followers did not recognize that the mother may well have been the main source of her unhappy feelings. In Freud's Dora case, the cause of her complaints and suffering – panic attacks, a nervous cough, and great aversion to, even revulsion of, anything sexual – remains unclear. Is it a case of a masturbation conflict, the traumatically experienced seduction by Mr K, or of sexual desires for Mr K and, initially, as a little girl, for the father? Other case descriptions by Freud concerning the female Oedipus complex are not available, which makes one suspect that he may already have doubted whether in the case of female development his oedipal theory worked fully.

Once Freud thought he had found what he was looking for – namely, the central importance of the child's love for the parent of the opposite sex, of the fantasies and sexual yearnings summarized as the Oedipus complex – he only wanted to see his hypothesis confirmed. This was partly the reason why he had less tolerance for listening to the patient without prejudice than he had when he was still working with Breuer. Because of the increasing emphasis on sexuality and in spite of the rejection of hypnosis, Freud's method grew to be more suggestive and more coercive. He could barely contain his anger about Dora's tendency to render him powerless – which he saw as her hysterical need for control. In the end, the treatment was terminated prematurely by Dora. Nevertheless, Freud's description of the transference and mutual seduction in the interaction with this intangible and misunderstood girl forms a marvellous reflection of all the elements that play a role in the concept of hysteria, which is as mysterious as ever. The story still reads as a novel.

Fantasies around the parent of the opposite sex in Freud's self-analysis had led him to the discovery of the male Oedipus complex (to which he did not give this name until much later on). During the Dora period he was trying to work this theory out for her. Freud continued to pursue the task of harmonizing female development with the little boy's Oedipus complex, which he had declared to be generally valid. Only at the end of his life did Freud discover the importance of the mother as a figure central to a girl's life. Therein Freud's blind spot for the role of mothers, first of all his own mother, who was an extremely dominant presence in his life, was playing tricks on him. For a long time, this hampered an insight into the development of girls and, less important here, into the origin of perversion in boys in which the mother tends to play an equally central role.[23]

Hysteria after *Studies on Hysteria*

Around 1900 Sigmund Freud's interest in hysteria was beginning to wane. Perhaps he was growing somewhat tired of his difficult patients. Be that as it may, besides on the phobia of Little Hans, Freud published no more than a few short articles and scattered comments on the topic. A cohesive theory on hysteria that might replace the survey in *Studies* never did appear.[24] This work continued to be the foundation for the understanding of hysterical psychological functioning, both in Freud's self-analysis and in his analysis of his patients.

Freud's quest for the source of hysteria as prototype of neurosis – his most important subject from his *Studies* up to and including Dora – put him on the track of psychoanalysis. On the basis of his studies on hysteria he discovered the laws of unconscious thinking. The laws underlying the formation of symptoms are similar to thought processes seen in dreams – for example, dreams make use of displacement and condensation: one person can stand for another person, a fact or image or individual can stand for several facts, images, or individuals. *'Fehlleistungen'*, or so-called errors, not to mention the joke and the sources of humour, became comprehensible and meaningful instead of arbitrary and pointless. To his female hysteria patients Freud also owed the formulation of phenomena such as repression, transference, and defence.

Revolutions can go too far, whereupon restoration generally follows. The same thing happened to Freud's ideas about the all-encompassing sexuality and the Oedipus complex that he developed after the *Studies on Hysteria*. Generalizing on the basis of one single idea, as Freud did, was common in the nineteenth century but has, since then, been superseded. What is all the more remarkable is that many of Freud's early ideas have come back, and some have even turned out to be more useful than his more generalized, later theory. According to some authors, the early Freud is more frequently right than the later one.[25]

These days, hysterical characteristics are no longer seen as separate from the interaction with parents, such as seduction in the sense of prematurely aroused desires, which have more to do with the needs of the adult than those of the child. The mother's role, which Freud did not connect with hysteria, has been studied in greater depth since then. Not until the end of his life did Freud mention the mother's seduction of the child, specifically in connection with the mother–daughter relationship and female sexuality.

Many hastily developed concepts from the early days of psychoanalysis – such as hypnosis, trauma, seduction – that had rapidly faded into the background, are now receiving full attention again. Posttraumatic stress syndrome is a diagnosis that is frequently made today. Similarly, there is renewed interest in child abuse, sexual exploitation, and incest. The currently prevailing therapy using hypnosis, known as hypnotherapy, is a modern version of the old method used by Breuer and Freud. Catharsis was metamorphosed into primal-scream therapy by the American psychologist Arthur Janov and experienced by John Lennon, who recorded it. The concept of consciousness splitting is now generally accepted, not only in psychoanalysis but in general psychiatry as well. Dissociative disorder, an old diagnosis from the *Studies*, is now popularly known as multiple personality disorder. In this connection the term dissociation is used, a more rigorous form of repression, as a defence against serious traumas.

'Does hysteria exist?' is a question that continues to be posed. Nevertheless, anxiety hysteria, the state of being phobically or diffusely fearful – a term introduced by Freud's Viennese contemporary Wilhelm Stekel[26] – is still the most widespread neurosis. In children, having all sorts of fears – fear of the dark, fear of being left alone – is actually a normal and passing condition. Children's fears do not indicate a disorder, unless they are vehement and long-lasting, in which case they do connote future problems. Conversion hysteria – converting emotional problems into physical symptoms – is and remains the prototype and first form of neurosis because body language is the first language. Aside from the encyclopaedia of the 1950s,[27] now out-dated, by the American psychoanalyst Otto Fenichel, who distinguishes between anxiety hysteria, phobia, and conversion, and the hysterical character of Wilhelm Reich,[28] one of Freud's students, post-Freudian psychoanalytic literature has produced only a few fundamental or new ideas about hysteria. Initially all hysteria was conversion. In the 1950s, the American psychoanalyst Otto Rangell rightfully determined that conversion and hysteria can appear separately and that therefore the two are definitely not synonymous.[29]

In the meantime, hysteria has not vanished from the clinics in the least. Verbally less developed people, in particular, still tend to express emotional conflicts by physical means. The offices of physicians are still full of patients with conversion symptoms. Psychiatrists are visited by people with every possible complaint of a hysterical nature. Psychiatric clinics are populated, among others, with children, adolescents, and adults with hysterical psychoses.

The description of what hysteria includes and its explanation follows on the heels of psychoanalytic theory and changes accordingly. The origin of hysteria has now more generally shifted to early childhood. A lack of a sense of basic security is more important than oedipal yearnings, sexuality is less important than a solid feeling of self-worth. Conflicts from early life, such as oral-sadistic conflicts (around weaning, eating and refusing food, poisoning and being poisoned) and anal-sadistic strivings (soiling, stubborn resistance, pinching off) are strongly represented. Both aggression and guilt are strongly repressed and preferably projected onto the other person. Passivity, helplessness, and seductiveness are part of the core of hysteria.

In the meantime, the hysteria of early psychoanalysis that was allegedly easy to treat is now more often designated as a hard-to-cure archaic disorder.[30] Eroticizing seductive behaviour (especially of women) appears to be pseudo-sexuality that originates from a need to please and in so doing to become loved. It points to early problems that resulted in a weak sense of self-worth. In that case, erotic seduction must serve to erase that insecurity and to make the other person now love the insecure individual. It has little to do with eroticism, and the suggestion does not cover the overtones.

The English psychoanalyst Eric Brenman came up with the cryptic phrase: 'Although I do not know what the word hysteric means, I do know it when I meet one.'[31] He then relates the story of a man who manipulates him, renders him powerless, and wants him to believe in a phantom reality. That hysteria does appear in men as well was already a known fact at the end of the nineteenth century, with the common example being the figure of Don Juan. This is a man who must compulsively and constantly prove his manhood.

Even today no one is yet capable of defining exactly what hysteria consists of as emotional disorder. In the DSM–IV (the psychiatric diagnostic manual, according to which each disorder must be labelled) this diagnosis is missing or, rather, is replaced by the 'dissociative' or 'histrionic' personality disorder. A new historic study on the subject calls it a 'state of mind'.[32]

Fantasy and reality

The primary problem with which Sigmund Freud struggled has yet to be resolved. How can the therapist decide – when a memory is reconstructed during treatment – whether this is a case of fantasy or of reality? After all, a life story is neither one nor the other but, rather, a combination of the two. Reconstruction of the past as an intermediary step is inescapable for almost every memory. Every life story is situated within the force field of fantasy and reality. Today, reconstruction of early life history is almost abandoned as a method. The relationship of analyst and patient in the here and now is considered most revealing of present and early perceptual distortions.

For a long time psychoanalysis would not hear of psychic traumas caused by social terror or private violence. For all too long, the complaints of persecution survivors who had been threatened with extermination were seen as the results of disorders stemming from early childhood.[33] Child abuse, sexual exploitation, and incest were often disregarded.[34]

Currently one can find excesses in the opposite direction: therapists who talk their clients into 'repressed' memories of sexual abuse. They go back to Freud's pre-1897 seduction theory and explain every disorder on the basis of sexual trauma, ignoring his warning that it often concerns fantasies. These 'recovered memory' or 'repressed memory' therapists, who occupy themselves with the tracing of forgotten memories, frequently find facts that have never actually happened.[35] This gives rise to all sorts of unpalatable accusations, many of them without any foundation. They make the question whether a trauma has to do with a real memory or a fantasy relevant once again. In reaction to the suggestive techniques they apply, which can create major damage, research has been done that hopes to demonstrate that repression does not exist.[36] An often vicious discussion has erupted around the 'false memory' syndrome – memories that turn out not to be memories but are based on the therapist's suggestion. Here are cited the early Freud and traumas that, according to him, are repressed. Presumably he, too, suggested too much to his patients. Furthermore, the later Freud is vilified because he should never have abandoned the seduction theory.[37]

Some critics use the 'repressed and recovered' therapists as living proof that Freud supposedly talked his patients into a sexual trauma, just as they do. Others, the Swiss psychoanalyst Alice Miller[38] and the controversial publicist Jeffrey Moussaief Masson[39] among them, claim that Freud abandoned his seduction theory against his own better knowledge.

Hysteria today

The London psychoanalyst Eric Brenman mentions four aspects of hysteria: the denial of both internal and external reality, the tendency to convince the other person that one is right, fleeting identifications with some idol or other, and a possessive dependency. Hysteria is based on 'wishful thinking', on unrealistic delusions.[40] Manipulation and attempts at intruding into the thoughts and feelings of the other person serve to make the other believe in a non-existent reality and to suggest highly dramatic events. A catastrophe is feared – which must be withstood through fear, phobia, or conversion – and, at the same time, the person denies that anything is wrong. Specifically, the almost manic mood and the unfounded excitement serve to keep a depression, often hidden behind hysteria, under control. The vehemence conceals a sense of emptiness created by splitting and repression (dissociation) of undesirable fantasies.

Symptoms such as fierce and persistent (transference) love for the therapist have to do with repairing a narcissistic lack: 'Love me', is the message. The fear of not being attractive and not being sexually pleasing plays a major role. Attempts at seduction are made without acting upon them because they have little or nothing to do with sexuality. Frigidity may serve to deny sexuality, while its opposite, preoccupation with sexuality, may serve to disavow sexual problems and victimization to deny aggression. As previously mentioned, feelings of insufficiency in so-called eroticizing patients often have to do with a seductive parent whose desires the child could not possibly satisfy.

Concerning the origin of hysteria, Brenman mentions several characteristics of the mother–child relationship: the mother is nervous and fears catastrophes; she suggests that she has the right solution for everything, thus offering the child no sense of reality and no realistic identification object. She stimulates denial of the child's inner experience of what is true and what is not. She provides it with idealizing, extolling, unreal love and titillates it with sensual satisfaction, whereby she kindles hyper-sexuality and dependency.

Today it is generally accepted that hysteria has more to do with a defence against depression, fear of abandonment, and a threatened sense of self-worth than with sexuality. Neither conversions nor any other physical or non-physical symptoms are conditions for being able to speak of hysteria. It is frequently related to an attitude to life, to character, more than to a circumscribed symptom. Several authors mention the aspect of remaining stuck in a childlike omnipotent fantasy of bisexuality. The desire to belong to both genders simultaneously has not been overcome. The same holds true for the denial of sexual difference, the difference between generations and that between subject and object. The boundaries between ego and non-ego can readily dissolve. For both men and women, fixation on a phallic level, the fantasy that having a penis, is essential for achieving happiness and fulfilment of every desire, and the accompanying increased fear of castration always play a role.

Fantasy has merely a symbolic function in hysteria and does not serve as preparation for realistic plans. It leads to plans that run aground halfway and do not attain any satisfaction. Out of fear of traumas being repeated, the person would rather seek active object loss (attracting and rejecting) than enter into a bond that could be broken again. Possessiveness and the need to intrude into the life of the other are denied and projected onto that other person: 'It is he who wants to meddle in my life, interfere with me, start a relationship with me, seduce me.'

Hysterical transference, for example, falling madly in love with the therapist, is just as unreal and seductive and often resembles quicksand. The unsolvable resentment and the irreparable deficiency that the therapist has to handle can summon up strongly negative countertransference feelings. Innocent, infantile, sometimes sadomasochistic accusations can arouse feelings of antipathy.

The hysterical personality hides his longing for admiring love behind the superficiality of his relationships and identifies with the fascinated spectator of the drama he performs. Another characteristic is the cognitive style shown in observation, thinking, and consciousness. Repression, dissociation, and splitting may be categorized under the cognitive styles of hysteria. Sigmund Freud globally divided human types, distinguishing between the more compulsive and the more hysterical types. This division is still useful and reflects a distinction between the sexes as well. More often than not, the former – the compulsives or compulsive neurotics – are male, while those who tend towards hysteria are more often female.

The cognitive styles of the two types are different. Compulsive people tend to observe and remember and to report the facts with precision, albeit without the corresponding feelings. More hysterical character types have a tendency to forget, to keep everything vague; they readily mystify, or they imagine all kinds of things that never happened (fabrication); they are less observant, and they have more gaps in their story, which is draped in feelings that may give the impression of being exaggerated and artificial.

Finally, another characteristic may emerge – that is, identification as a means of relating to the other person and by doing so filling and covering up one's own vacuum. The hysterical personality identifies as effortlessly and as superficially with living people as with fantasy objects such as movie stars and athletic heroes. Via his fantasy about others he experiences what was lost in his personal inner life through repression. Empathy with the other as a separate and independent person is often lacking.

Projective identification – experiencing via the other what is suppressed in one's own inner life – serves to combat insecurity and feelings of insufficiency. 'He is in love with me, I don't find him attractive.' This often has to do with rapidly reversible and fleeting crushes – quick idealization of someone, disappointment in that person, then repeating the same process all over again with someone else. The hysterical personality will try to discard fears by projecting them onto the object and then identifying with him from afar. This may occur, for example, by rendering the other powerless and insecure, whereby these feelings are shifted from subject to object. Josef Breuer experienced the chaos and despair that the hysterical personality can incite in the partner with Anna O, who reigned over him through her illness and helplessness, leading him up the garden path.

We are all familiar with 'shopping' – running from one therapist to another – behaviour that several patients in the *Studies* demonstrated. The care provider is first encountered with an idealizing attitude, is then found to be disappointing, is subsequently vilified, and is finally dumped.

Hysteria and the woman

Bisexual aspirations, the desire to be both male and female, continue to feature with undiminished force in Sigmund Freud's later publications on hysteria.[41]

A girl is not the ideal object of her mother who often prefers the little boy, and she is too small to excite her father. This is why she would most like to be both boy and girl at the same time. First she has to try to play up to her mother, later her father, and thus she might be rejected twice. She learns early to please, to show off, to pretend to be different from what she really is. She is more often insecure about her body, her worth as a person, and her ability to hold the other person's attention. She mobilizes her erotic appeal to yet acquire what she did not automatically receive. She offers herself as an object of delight for the other's pleasure, thereby to gain love and prop up her sense of self-worth.

Of course, all these factors were far more applicable in the bygone Victorian era than is now the case. However, there will always be consequences attached to the state of being male or female. After all, being born to a mother as either a boy or a girl, the gender, the development of the two sexes is different and not a mirror image, one of the other. The woman has a special relationship with her body because of her constantly changing physical situation. Her menstruating, pregnant, menopausal ever-changeable body, her physical structure with internal, invisible sexual organs, can all be a factor in the more frequent appearance of hysteria in women. The already mentioned cognitive characteristics of hysteria that play a role in both genders are, incidentally, maintaining vagueness in observation and keeping the story unclear. This vagueness in the world of representation is reinforced because woman's experience of sexuality is more diffuse and can be less clearly localized than that of the man.

The man, on the other hand, has a hard time identifying with the complete sexual and emotional abandonment of which the woman is capable. Normally speaking, her sexual experience is less focused on the sex organ and on

performance than on the internal experience. Desire for fusion and abandonment of control are more characteristic of the female.

Both male and female hysteria have to do with the lack of a conception
(or with the denial) of female gender. Gender difference is blurred, and one
pretends that there is just one gender, the male. This is one of the reasons why
sexuality continues to be heavily phallic in colour, expressed in a desire to be
noticed, in provocation and assertiveness as a stereotypical sign of success.
In hysteria, both in men and women, the pseudo-male and pseudo-female
that feels artificial replaces passivity and dependency as a defence against
that feared and rejected femininity. What plays a role in both sexes is an
unconscious resistance against an overly strong identification with the wishes
of the problematic mother figure. This is the opposite of the symbiotic illusion
where the desire to please the mother is given free rein.

Woman and her body

There are several reasons for greater narcissistic sensitivity and a vulnerable
sense of self-worth in women.

First of all, the female body, more than that of the male, is an emotional
battleground and a source of concern because of the constant and always
returning hormonal changes and variations. This makes women's narcissism
around the body more vulnerable than that of men.

Second, a girl must first please her mother, her first love object, her first
partner of the same sex, her lifelong example. Somewhat later she also wishes
to capture her father's love and attention. She can certainly succeed in both
ventures, but she also runs the risk of a double disappointment. Furthermore,
her hetero- and homosexual aspirations lead to a reinforced bisexuality, in
the double sense of wanting to be both masculine and feminine and yearning
for both male and female love.

Third, a girl runs the risk of maintaining a close symbiotic bond with the
mother and not becoming independent from her, which will affect her sense
of self-worth.

All these factors put together, plus the fact that a girl is usually less focused
on sexuality than a boy and needs more time to learn to enjoy her own body,
may incite her to behave in a quasi-sexual, seductive manner. When the need
for love and attention is disguised as sexuality, it can be called a hysterical
character trait. Her quest for narcissistic support can readily take the form
of wanting to please and do favours for others, which will make her more
inclined to behave in a theatrical and non-authentic fashion. Since she pays
close attention to her physical changes and functions, she is more attuned to
physical feelings and more inclined to have imaginary physical sensations or
develop hypochondriacal fears.

Women often choose body language over verbalization so that their desires
remain concealed, which is what made Sigmund Freud exclaim: 'What does

woman want?' Actually, she herself often does not know. In the nineteenth century women had few means at their disposal to make hidden yearnings known, other than fainting or some other physical symptoms. This was known as conversion – what we call somatization today – and was classified under the label hysteria. As a diagnosis this is far too limited because the various manifestations of hysteria are culturally determined. 'Hysteria is a mimetic disorder: it is an imitation of culturally permitted expressions of disgust or suffering.'[42] In the nineteenth century it was fainting, something we would see as highly transparent today. Chronic fatigue is currently much more accepted as an expression of discomfort.

Hysteria, in the more limited sense of a physical expression of emotional turmoil, continues to be the prototype and the earliest form of neurosis, just as body language is the baby's first language. In the case of the girl, such body language will continue to be important.

The girl's psychological equilibrium will be sorely tested for the first time during puberty, a period when new impulses such as sexual drives will require her attention. The physical changes that then make their presence known may arouse fear and shame instead of pride. Her shape and silhouette change when her breasts begin to grow, which were not there before, and she must adjust her self-image accordingly. She must also accept her menstruation as a definitive change, for thereafter she will always experience monthly variations in her body and psyche. She can no longer pretend to have a choice about being boy or girl (although the unconscious fantasy that she has a choice may continue to be present, a phenomenon that I have encountered frequently both in pre- and post-menopausal women).

The body of a girl changes so much that she becomes attractive to men before she is aware of what is going on. Boys of the same age seem younger to her, she does not receive much interest from them, nor is she especially interested in them, but adult men suddenly seem to take a fancy to her. If the girl is not ready to handle this change, it can be terrifying because her internal experience of herself is so totally different from her external appearance. Moreover, she is lacking in the experience of being penetrated, even if she masturbates, which is not always the case. It is like Brünhilde, Richard Wagner's heroine in *Siegfried*, who exclaims:

'Wehe! Wehe! Wehe der Schmach, der schmächlichen Not! Verwundet hat mich, der mich erweckt! Er erbrach mir Brünne und Helm: Brünhilde bin ich nicht mehr!' '. . . aus Nebel und Grau'n windet sich wütend ein Angstgewirr: Schrecken schreitet und bäumt sich empor!'[43]

[Woe, woe, woe the insult, the shameful affliction! He who aroused me (my sexuality) has wounded me! He broke my coat of mail and my helmet: I am no longer Brünhilde!' '. . . out of fog and dusk a furious and terrifying chaos of fear emerges: terror strides and rears aloft.']

The girl, and later the woman, has little control over her unmanageable body, in which all kinds of things happen – invisible, hidden inside her. Fairly soon a continuous, uncontrollable physical and psychological process of change begins to which she must grow accustomed. All of the above make mood changes in the girl almost inevitable.

It is impossible to return to a previous state. Looking back is risky, just as it was for Lot's wife, who was turned into a pillar of salt when she looked back at Sodom.

By not eating, the anorexic girl protests against the unstoppable processes in her body, which point irrevocably to gender identity and sexuality. She can put a stop to menstruation this way, thereby reducing her fertility to zero. She can refuse the feminine role, evade encounters with the other sex, be active in athletics until she drops, and become as muscular as a boy. However, all of that does mean regression.

Menstruation is followed by a transition: that from innocent girl to moody adolescent. After her first period, she becomes an 'immaculate' albeit sexually mature virgin. As mentioned before, hereafter the monthly return of sensations in her body make the girl more sensitive to signs of physical well-being and to conversion – that is, for expressing emotions via the body. Perhaps she previously was a tomboy who had not yet chosen whether she wanted to be a boy or a girl. She thought she still had both options open. Now she has to be a woman, whether she likes it or not. For girls the development of a healthy narcissism, a healthy sense of self-worth, and a healthy pride in being-woman are frequently threatened by too many factors to make it through unscathed.

Menstruation increases the girl's bewilderment with her female genitals. Because she has absolutely no control over them, the girl is thrown back onto her old fears from the time that her anus and vagina were confused. Her cloaca fantasies – the childhood idea that one opening serves various purposes, from fertilization via procreation to elimination – are experienced anew, which may lead to an aversion to her own body. It is sometimes difficult for a girl not to see her body as unattractive, dirty, and contemptible. She must resist feelings of shame. Of course, a mother can help her daughter to develop a different view of herself. Regular conversations about the body and sexual functions can become a source of insight and emancipation for the girl. The mother's positive contribution depends on the extent to which she herself is able to discuss bodily functions and physical sensations without showing any signs of inner conflicts on the topic.

However, the girl's body image is sometimes weighed down by taboos and archaic fantasies, such as destroying and being destroyed by the mother. This will make her more inclined to a lack of self-assurance and disgust with her body rather than contentment with her womanhood. She thinks that she is dirty and contagious, that she is ugly or mean, that she is as dangerous as a vampire – or else that she is being threatened by the hatred of a malevolent mother. All one needs to do is remember the grandmother–wolf who devours Little Red Riding Hood or the stepmother who poisons Snow White.

Later on, during adolescence, a girl can develop self-assurance and pride in her looks, can spruce herself up, go out, and notice what effect she has on people. This is an experimental phase in which future roles are tested. She attracts and rejects male attention, which can still be as feared and desired as before.

When a girl has her first sexual experience, no matter how exciting it may have been, something is lost for her, too, because she has been changed from virgin to woman. Once deflowered, never a virgin again. And that is merely the beginning of all the changes, not the end. In the West, a girl generally does not marry at a young age and does not want to become pregnant right away. For a long time she must be capable of taking measures to manage her sex life and protect herself from undesired pregnancies and sexually transmitted diseases such as chlamydia. However, the fact that procreation is possible in principle triggers longings, fears, and fantasies with regard to fertility and infertility, as well as ambivalence around the desire to have or not have any children. But the biological clock keeps ticking, and, unfortunately, for women the time to make exceedingly important decisions is limited.

If the girl wants children, she must decide whether she wants to enter into a steady relationship with a male partner. If everything goes according to plan, the woman will become pregnant when she wishes it – an experience that may be a new source of concern and fear. Even though she wanted it, once she is pregnant she often feels trapped because once again she has lost her options to choose: she cannot change her mind. She will never again *not* be a mother. Because she is gaining weight, she often fears she can no longer compete with other women. She begins to be afraid that her partner will no longer find her attractive, will start looking at other women, be unfaithful.

I have noticed that many a young expectant mother goes through an episode in which she falls in love with the first man who happens to cross her path, as an escape from her recently created cage. But even when she does not go to such extremes, she definitely has mixed feelings of both joy and regret, because she will never again be a free woman without lifelong responsibilities.

Every choice has its disadvantages. If she has no children, it is equally inevitable that she will regret not having a family later on, even if the decision was consciously made. Once a family has been formed, however, the train inexorably rushes on towards middle age, the time that children leave home, the inescapable phase of menopause that finally culminates in the spectre of old age. The fear of no longer being physically attractive is a typical female complaint that is wholly connected to the body and its whims.

A girl's or woman's sexuality can be repressed together with her appetite, which may lead to anorexia nervosa, a reaction that closely resembles hysteria because of the accompanying false body image and the rejection of sexuality, the need for attention, the theatricality, and the narcissistic vulnerability. A disorder such as anorexia might be linked to a girl's desperate attempts to control the uncontrollable changes in her body and to remain a bisexual or asexual boyish girl. The extremely important, emotionally laden steps and phases that her body encounters could cause frigidity in the girl.

As a rule a girl's first sexual experiences are more frightening than pleasurable. It may take a long time before a woman learns what pleases her and imparts her wishes, which for so long had been unknown or concealed to herself. It can even take a very long time for her to have her first orgasm, to finally discover her body's possibilities, and to know how to share those with a partner. One can only hope that twenty-first-century mothers will find it less difficult to discuss the body and sexual or erotic feelings so that daughters will no longer have to figure out how to get the necessary information from their girlfriends.

For women, eroticism is more complicated and emotionally charged than for men. During adolescence girls are already more aware than boys that sexuality has two aspects: procreation and eroticism. She can become pregnant, the boy cannot. For the sexually mature girl the clitoris still has only one function: pleasure. For an inhibited girl or a nun this is, unlike the penis, a useless organ that may not be discovered or touched. On the other hand, in girls and women the multiple functions of the vagina can lead to confusion about their body. The vagina is a hollow organ: something, such as sperm or a penis, can be put inside or vanish there. It can also serve as an exit: for babies, for excretion, for menstrual blood. It is readily associated with pain but may also provide pleasure, usually after stimulation of the clitoris. Thus, there is a mysterious connection between those two organs. The woman must be able to distinguish between all these different functions and yet, at the same time, not lose sight of the connections. For the boy it is simpler: he has a single organ that does everything: urination, sex, and masturbation. Children do not come forth from it, and it has nothing to do with pain.

Lastly, something about the woman and her discontents. Girls and women are all too often unhappy with the way they look. If they are blonde, they want to be brunette. If they have curls, they want to have straight hair. If they are short, they want to be tall. And almost always they wish they were thinner. Generally something is missing that keeps them from being happy with what they are. When they think of themselves as really ugly, it often has little to do with their looks. That may be a translation in concrete physical terms of the view they have of themselves – namely, as 'bad' or 'reprehensible', that is to say jealous, hostile, with nasty thoughts and bitchy desires.

It may also be that in the family the space available for beauty is fully occupied by the mother, who is the only one with the privilege of being an attractive prima donna and admired as such by the father. She is the first lady, the pinnacle of femininity, the only one who possesses the secrets of charm. In that case, the girl automatically occupies the space left for her and becomes the ugly duckling, the Cinderella of the family. She loses her sense of self-worth and thinks: my mother is beautiful and attractive, I am not. Because she lacks self-esteem, she becomes dependent on the compliments and appreciation of others who have to constantly reassure her. This state of affairs renders women narcissistically vulnerable, something that every Casanova knows and exploits. However, a mother can strongly stimulate (or obstruct) her daughter's self-confidence. Some mothers praise their daughters, others criticize them in order to solidify their own vulnerable psychological equilibrium.

Female eroticism and excitement are experienced as more diffuse and less easy to locate than those of the male. This may have an influence on the girl's corporal experience. Her physical build influences her body-image and how she experiences her body-self. This representation influences her cognition, the way in which she perceives – not merely the way in which she perceives her own body, but also the way in which she perceives the world around her. Her perceptions tend to be less clear-cut and less sharply defined.

In my opinion, the specific characteristics of the woman play a role in the fact that hysteria appears more frequently in women than in men. The most important factor there is the very special relationship that the woman has with her continuously changing physical situation. In the field of psychoanalysis this aspect of femininity has never received the attention that it deserves. In addition to the constant exchange of feelings between mother and daughter, which binds them through thick and thin, the daughter also has to deal with the dramatic metamorphoses she herself undergoes.

How hysteria is expressed depends on time and place and follows upon the heels of the cultural process. In the old days a girl was said to be possessed of the devil and had to be exorcised. She was able to curve her back like a hoop, know as 'arc de cercle'. She might have a false pregnancy, become blind or paralysed. These days, all of this would be too transparent and lead to being called hysterical as a term of abuse. Today the hysteric may be attacked by 'enemy aliens', fall prey to mysterious exhaustion, develop indemonstrable backaches – all of these, as in earlier times, serving to escape from conflicts.

Still, the biological body is unalterable and of all time. The exceedingly important and emotionally laden steps and phases that her body has to confront may terrify a girl. She will be more inclined to see her body as a battlefield on which every emotional struggle has to be thrashed out. She has a greater tendency towards somatization than the boy – that is to say, towards converting psychological conflicts, problems, and distress into physical symptoms for which no physical cause can be found. She is tormented by headaches, abdominal pain, fatigue, and nausea. She suffers from all sorts of apparently inexplicable physical aches and pains that might be expressing her hidden erotic fantasies and preoccupations. Symptoms carry a meaning even when the person in question has no other than physical means by which to express or articulate her tensions.

The powerless therapist

The idea that hysteria no longer occurs is mistaken – nothing could be further from the truth. As mentioned before, both anxiety hysteria (diffuse fears) and conversions (physical complaints with psychological causes) are still prevalent among the less educated and the verbally less fluent. The more 'proto-professionalized' – that is, those who are quite aware of the now highly popularized psychoanalytic notions – use more subtle forms that are less transparent, such as creating dramas and horrors that have never happened. But dramatization and artificiality have existed since time immemorial. Hysteria follows along with time and place and culture. The same holds true for related symptoms, such as anorexia, by means of which one can also follow the psychological approach across the centuries.[44] Hysteria has the chameleon-like feature that it knows how to handle what the social environment or the therapist expects of it. These days it concerns more existential complaints, unease with existence, a diffuse discontent, and often vague complaints that are hard to classify as physical syndromes. Chronic fatigue syndrome may well belong here as a modern form of hysteria. What is more, no one needs to feel offended by this because hysteria is not an abusive term but a serious condition that in no way rests on affectation.

In practice, when it is misunderstood, hysteria is often misleading and renders one powerless because of the impossibility of a meaningful dialogue, at least on the level that the patient involuntarily indicates: adult eroticism. When a connection can be made with depression and a lack of self-esteem, entering into a conversation on the right level and avoiding eroticizing inter-action becomes more feasible. Denial of depression and denial of mourning are frequently mentioned as that which is missing in hysteria. Mourning the lost love object, namely the loss of the mother's or father's love, is often converted into artificial sexual excitement. The therapist must be able to resist the temptation to be swept along by that pseudo-sexual, pseudo-adult eroti-cism. It is better to hold on to the hypothesis that the patient's fears are being played out on a much more primitive level of experience.

Katherine

Katherine, one among many with similar complaints, is approaching fifty. She suffers from feelings of depression, violent migraines, hyperventilation, and panic attacks. She has been happily married for the past ten years or so, but when I ask her how she feels about not having any children she begins to sob. She is seeing me because she has heard that I am 'so great' and probably the 'only one who can help her'. I am the most recent one in a long series of physicians, physiotherapists, acupuncturists, and other caregivers.

Katherine is sweet, innocent, and seductive, but otherwise she has a rather passive attitude. She says that there is little she can say about herself, and she leaves it to me to come up with the right questions. After a few conversations I notice that I am busy making efforts on her behalf without much of a response other than the statement that so far it has not helped at all, and she has been in bed again for the entire week with dreadful headaches. In the end, I decide to suggest that she seems to find it rather pleasant to see me plod along without any result, and so I say: 'You are wearing a red scarf today, which gives me an idea. You are the bullfighter and I am the bull confronting a red piece of fabric that he is vainly attacking. He cannot win and finally has to be beaten by the bullfighter.' The image makes her laugh involuntarily. She senses very well what I talking about and secretly enjoys it. Her making me powerless leads back to her own feeling of powerlessness, her self-image of being without any talent, a failure, worthless. She would like to be 'intelligent', 'educated', and 'special'. She would like to be admired. Instead, she feels she is nothing.

As an obstinate adolescent who left home early, she missed out on almost any education. She had little guidance from her upwardly mobile and insecure parents. Nothing was ever discussed at home: exchanges with her mother – with whom she speaks almost daily – concern nothing but 'trivia'. She has 'never accomplished anything special', and she feels her childlessness as a miserable failure as well.

We explore what it is that Katherine would like to have been and like to have done. We more or less systematically work through the mourning over aging (see chapter 8) – the sorrow over all that is lost and will never come back, in the first place her own youth. For Katherine, the wish to acquire her own place in the world is linked to jealousy of her husband, a successful painter. She idealizes and admires him while she draws attention to herself by being ill.

After about three months of '*belle indifférence*' (an old-fashioned term for hysterical innocence and quasi-ignorance), traumatic memories of abortions she has had come to the surface. She presents vivid fantasies and dreams that contain a wealth of symbolism around fear and eroticism. Suddenly she has a lot to say, although this phase will turn out to be short-term.

All in all, aside from greater attention paid to the (negative) transference, the problems and the manner of treatment seem not to differ that much from the cases described in *Studies on Hysteria* and Dora.

In conclusion

In conclusion one may posit that great care is certainly required in using hysteria as a diagnosis. The *Studies* were created at a time when Sigmund Freud, leaving the tradition in psychiatry of classification and mere labelling of disorders, began to listen to his patients. 'Hysteria' can function as a caricature or as a term of abuse. Rejecting it may lead to denying the fact that there is no dearth of concrete examples in everyday practice. These days, the 'pure syndrome' that has never existed is supplemented by a more balanced diagnostic.

By studying the literature on hysteria and its history, one learns to look more closely. Phenomena that might be overlooked without this knowledge suddenly become recognizable and understandable. In the diagnostics of children, specifically, one can often identify a hysterical or compulsive neurotic character development early on, whereby treatment can be facilitated. The hysterical cognitive disposition is frequently recognizable in adults, even when the final diagnosis turns out to be a mixture of, or a different one from, hysteria. Over the last hundred years, the psychoanalyst's way of observing, as well as treatment technique, has been expanded and refined, and it has grown more subtle, especially by involving the therapist far more deeply. Nevertheless, we cannot completely erase a personality structure that we are wont to label as 'hysterical'. The original discoveries that Freud gained from hysteria are not only of great historic importance but also still provide us with the necessary clinical knowledge today.

In a number of ways, the *Studies* are closer to our time than Freud's later work is. No absolute pronouncements are made yet, the knowledge of sexual phases did not yet exist, nor did the Oedipus complex. Freud was still searching, as is once again the case for his heirs today, now that many psychoanalytic axioms about femininity are up in the air while the clinical facts remain.

Freud's warning to his fiancée – 'Without knowing the past one cannot know the present' – is as true for the theory as it is for the individual. In order to understand the development of psychoanalysis, it is necessary to study that centenarian from its beginnings. Psychoanalysis as theory and as science is shaken to its foundations today. A particular way of thinking and perceiving is perhaps the only thing that will survive of it in the long run. This psycho-analytic way of looking now was already fully present in the *Studies*.

Notes

I Love and hate between mothers and daughters

1 C. G. Jung invented the term Electra complex, and first mentioned it in his *Freud und die Psychoanalyse. Versuch einer Darstellung der psychoanalytischen Theorie. Gesammelte Werke*, Vol. 4, Olten, Walter Verlag 1971 [1913], pp. 107–230. However, he did not elaborate any further on the topic of specifically female development. Sigmund Freud rejected the term Electra complex – see also Daniel Dervin, 'The Electra complex: A history of misrepresentations', *Gender and Psychoanalysis* 4, 1998, 451–470. He, too, claims that no serious consideration was ever given to the Electra complex in connection with female development. For another author who favours the term Electra complex, see Doris Bernstein, *Female Identity Conflict in Clinical Practice*, Ed. N. Friedman & B. Distler, Northvale, NJ, Jason Aronson, 1993.

2 Daniel N. Stern, *The Motherhood Constellation: A Unified View of Parent–Infant Psychotherapy*, New York, Basic Books, 1995. Stern makes a careful exception to the Oedipus complex. He argues that around the time of pregnancy and delivery, the mother and grandmother of the woman and her child hold a far more central position than do her husband and her father. I agree with that, but in my opinion many more marginal notes concerning female development could be made with regard to the Oedipus complex.

2 The symbiotic illusion

1 Daniel N. Stern, *The Interpersonal World of the Infant: A View from Psychoanalysis and Developmental Psychology*, New York, Basic Books, 1985.

2 Perversions also appear in women, but they take a different form: for example, in an artificial show of super-femininity that is meant to hide other, often masculine, aspirations – see L. J. Kaplan, *Female Perversions*, London, Pandora Press, 1991.

3 M. S. Mahler, *On Human Symbiosis and the Vicissitudes of Individuation*, New York, International Universities Press, 1968.

4 M. S. Mahler, 'Aggression in the service of separation–individuation: Case study of a mother–daughter relationship', *Psychoanalytic Quarterly*, 50, 1981, 625–638.

5 M. S. Mahler, F. Pine, & A. Bergman, *The Psychological Birth of the Human Infant: Symbiosis and Individuation*, London, Hutchinson, 1975, chapter 10.

6 J. McDougall, 'Eve's reflection: On the homosexual components of female sexuality', in H. C. Meyers (Ed.), *Between Analyst and Patient: New Dimensions in Countertransference and Transference*, Hillsdale, NJ, The Analytic Press, 1986, pp. 213–228.

7 See, for example, T. B. Brazelton & B. Cramer, *The Earliest Relationship: Parents, Infants and the Drama of Early Attachment*, London, Karnac Books, 1991; P. Fonagy & M. Target, 'Playing with reality I: Theory of mind and the normal development of psychic reality', *International Journal of Psycho-Analysis*, 77, 2, 1996, 217–235; S. Lebovici, *Le Nourisson, la mère et le psychanalyste: Les interactions précoces*, Paris, Paidos le Centurion, 1983.

8 M. M. Khan, 'The role of polymorph-perverse body experiences and object-relations in ego-integration', 1962, in C. Yorke (Ed.), *Alienation in Perversions*, London, The Hogarth Press, 1979, pp. 31–55.

9 H. C. Halberstadt-Freud, 'Clara Schumann: "A woman's love and life: A psychoanalytic interpretation"', *The Psychohistory Review*, 23, 2, Winter 1995, 143–166.

10 Helene Deutsch, *The Psychology of Women: A Psychoanalytic Interpretation*, Vol. I, New York, Grune & Stratton, 1944; Helene Deutsch, *The Psychology of Women: A Psychoanalytic Interpretation*, Vol. II, New York, Grune & Stratton, 1945.

3 History of maternal love

1 H. P. Blum, 'The maternal ego-ideal and the regulation of maternal qualities', in G. H. Pollock & S. I. Greenspan (Eds.), *The Course of Life, Psychoanalytic Contributions towards Understanding Personality Development*, Vol. III, *Adulthood and the Aging Process*, Adelphi, MA, Mental Health Study Center, 1981, pp. 91–114.

2 C. Lasch, *Haven in a Heartless World: The Family Besieged*, New York, Basic Books, 1975.

3 See, among others, P. Ariès, *L'enfant et la vie familiale sous l'ancien régime*, Paris, Seuil, 1973; E. Badinter, *L'amour en plus: Histoire de l'amour maternel* (*XVIIe–XXe siècle*), Paris, Flammarion, 1980; A. Dally, *Inventing Motherhood: The Consequences of an Ideal*, London, Burnett, 1982; B. Harris, 'Two lives, one 24-hour day', in A. Roland & B. Harris (Eds.), *Career and Motherhood: Struggles for a New Identity*, New York, Human Sciences Press, 1979, pp. 24–45.

4 J. Donzelot, *La police des familles*, Paris, Editions de Minuit, 1977; M. Foucault, *Histoire de la folie*, Paris, Plon, 1961; M. Schatzman, *Soul Murder: Persecution in the Family*, London, Penguin, 1973; J. M. W. van Ussel, *De geschiedenis van het sexuele problem* [The history of the sexual problem], Meppel, Boom, 1982.

5 J. Bowlby, *Maternal Care and Mental Health*, Geneva, World Health Organization, 1951; A. Freud, *Infants without Families: Report on the Hampstead Nurseries 1939–1945*, New York, International Universities Press, 1973; H. Nagera, *Early Childhood Disturbances, the Infantile Neurosis, and the Adulthood Disturbances*, New York, International Universities Press, 1966; R. Spitz, 'Hospitalism. An inquiry into the genesis of psychiatric conditions in early childhood', *Psychoanalytic Study of the Child* 1, 1945, 53–74.

6 Ariès, 1973 (see note 3); D. Haks, *Huwelijk en gezin in Holland in de 17e en 18e eeuw* [Marriage and family in Holland in the seventeenth and eighteenth centuries], Assen, Van Gorcum, 1982; P. Laslett, *The World We Have Lost*, London, Methuen, 1965; P. Laslett, *Family Life and Illicit Love in Earlier Generations: Essays in Historical Sociology*, Cambridge, Cambridge University Press, 1977; L. deMause (Ed.), *The History of Childhood*, New York, Harper, 1974; E. Shorter, *The Making of the Modern Family*, Glasgow, Fontana Collins, 1975; L. Stone, *The Family, Sex and Marriage in England 1500–1800*, London, Penguin, 1977.

7 E. Le Roy Ladurie, *Montaillou: Village occitan de 1294 à 1324*, Paris, Gallimard, 1984.

8 P. Richier & D. Alexandre-Bidon, *L'enfance au moyen âge*, Paris, Seuil, 1994; W. Frijhoff, 'Impasses en beloften van de mentaliteitsgeschiedenis', *Tijdschrift voor Sociale Geschiedenis* 10, 1984, 406–437.

9 Under the leadership of Peter Laslett (1965, see note 6), and Alan MacFarlane and cited by Hugh Cunningham, *Children and Childhood in Western Society since 1500*, London/New York, Longman, 1995.

10 deMause, 1974 (see note 6).

11 J. Boswell, *The Kindness of Strangers: The Abandonment of Children in Western Europe from Late Antiquity to the Renaissance*, New York, Vintage Books, 1990.

12 Cunningham, 1995 (see note 9).

13 W. A. Mozart, *Briefe*, Zurich, Willi Reich, Menasse, 1948.

14 Saint Augustine, *Confessions*, Harmondsworth, UK, Penguin, 1961.

15 A. MacFarlane, *The Origins of English Individualism*, Oxford, Basil Blackwell, 1978.

16 I. Origo, *The Merchant of Prato: Daily Life in a Medieval Italian City*, Harmondsworth, UK, Penguin, 1963.

17 J. Héroard, 'Extraits du Journal d'Héroard (1601–1628) sur l'enfance et la jeunesse de Louis XIII', *Nouvelle Revue de Psychanalyse* 19, 1979, 268–330.

18 S. Freud, 'Psychoanalytic remarks on an autobiographically described case of paranoia (Dementia paranoides) ["The Schreber case"] [1911], *The Standard Edition of the Complete Psychological Works of Sigmund Freud* [henceforth *S. E.*], Vol. XII, London, The Hogarth Press, 1971, pp. 9–80.

19 Schatzman, 1973 (see note 4).

20 Ariès, 1973 (see note 3); Richier & Alexandre-Bidon, 1994 (see note 8); Shorter, 1975 (see note 6); Stone, 1977 (see note 6); Van Ussel, 1982 (see note 4).

21 N. Elias, *The Civilizing Process: Sociogenetic and Psychogenetic Investigations*, rev. ed., Oxford, Blackwell, 1994.

22 J. Huizinga, *Herfsttij der middeleeuwen* [Autumn of the Middle Ages], Amsterdam, Contact, 1999.

23 Haks, 1982, Stone, 1977, Shorter, 1975 (see note 6); S. Schama, *The Embarrassment of Riches: An Interpretation of Dutch Culture in the Golden Age*, London, Fontana Press, 1987; *Kinderen van alle tijden* [Children through the ages], Zwolle, Waanders, Catalogue North-Brabants Museum 's-Hertogenbosch, 1997.

24 See MacFarlane, 1978 (see note 15).

25 D. Riesman, *The Lonely Crowd*, New Haven, CT, Yale University Press, 1950.

26 D. de Rougemont, *L'amour et l'occident*, Paris, Plon, 1939.

27 Y. A. Verdoorn, *Volksgezondheid en sociale ontwikkeling: Beschouwingen over het gezondheidswezen te Amsterdam in de 19e eeuw* [Public health and social development. Observations on healthcare in Amsterdam in the nineteenth century], Utrecht, Aula Spectrum, 1965.

28 J. M. Masson (Ed.), *The Complete Letters of Sigmund Freud to Wilhelm Fliess, 1887–1904*, Cambridge, MA/London, The Belknap Press of Harvard University Press, 1985.

29 S. Freud, 'Analysis of a phobia in a five-year-old boy' [1909], *S. E.*, Vol. X, pp. 5–148.

30 S. Freud, 'A case of hysteria' [1905], *S. E.*, Vol. VII, pp. 7–112; S. Freud, 'Upon a case of obsessional neurosis' [1909], *S. E.*, Vol. X, pp. 153–25; S. Freud, 'From the history of an infantile neurosis' [1918], *S. E.*, Vol. XVII, pp. 7–123.

31 E. V. Welldon, *Mother, Madonna, Whore: The Idealization and Denigration of Motherhood*, London, Heinemann, 1989.

32 P. Ariès, 'Entretien', *Nouvelle Revue de Psychanalyse, L'enfant*, 19, 1979, 13–26.

33 Lasch, 1975 (see note 2).

34 I. Freud, *Mannen en moeders. De levenslange worsteling van zonen met hun moeders* [Men and mothers. The lifelong struggle of sons and their mothers], Amsterdam, Van Gennep, 2002. In this book I put the emphasis on the mother–son relationship in connection with homosexuality and perversions, where matricide plays a greater role than does patricide.

35 P. Blos, *Son and Father*, London, The Free Press, 1985; N. Chodorow, *The Reproduction of Mothering: Psychoanalysis and the Sociology of Gender*, Berkeley, University of California Press, 1978.

36 D. W. Winnicott, 'Ego distortion in terms of true and false self', in *The Maturational Process and the Facilitating Environment*, London, The Hogarth Press, 1972.

37 A. Mitscherlich & Eric Mosbacher *Society without the Father: A Contribution to Social Psychology*, Kindle Edition, 1992.

4 Nina: Daughter of a single mother

1 P. Blos, 'The second individuation process of adolescence', *Psychoanalytic Study of the Child*, 22, 1967, 162–187.

5 Electra versus Oedipus

1 S. Freud, 'Female sexuality' [1931], *S. E.*, Vol. XXI, pp. 223–243.

2 Both the Oedipus and the Electra complex continue to be a template. The development of heterosexuality and homosexuality is too varied and too complex to justify generalization in individual cases. N. Chodorow, 'Heterosexuality as a compromise formation: Reflections on the psycho-analytic theory of sexual development', *Psychoanalysis and Contemporary Thought*, 15, 1992, 267–302; N. Chodorow, *Femininities, Masculinities, Sexualities: Freud and Beyond*, London, Free Association Books, 1994; J. McDougall, *The Many Faces of Eros: A Psychoanalytic Exploration of Human Sexuality*, New York/London, Norton, 1995.

3 R. H. Balsam, 'The mother within the mother', *Psychoanalytic Quarterly*, 69, 2000, 465–492.

4 B. P. Bernstein, 'Mothers and daughters from today's psychoanalytic perspective', *Psychoanalytic Inquiry*, 24, 2004, 601–628.

5 Aeschylus, *Oresteia: Agamemnon*, tr. Robert Fagles, Harmondsworth, UK, Penguin, 1977; Sophocles, *Electra and Other Plays*, tr. E. F. Watling, Harmondsworth, UK, Viking/Penguin, 1953; Euripides, *Electra and other Plays*, tr. Richard Rutherford & John Davie, Harmondsworth, UK, Penguin, 1999; J. Giraudoux, *Electre*, Paris, Grasset, 1937; H. von Hofmannsthal, *Electra*, London, Boosey & Hawkes, 1908; E. O'Neill, *Mourning Becomes Electra* [1932], London, Jonathan Cape, 1984.

6 P. Grimal, *Dictionary of Classical Mythology*, Oxford/New York, Blackwell Reference, 1986.

7 Freud, 'Female sexuality' [1931] (see note 1).

8 S. Freud, 'Fragment of an analysis of a case of hysteria' [1905], *S. E.*, Vol. VII, pp. 3–122.

9 R. B. Blass, 'Did Dora have an Oedipus complex? A re-examination of the theoretical context of Freud's "Fragments of an analysis" ', *Psychoanalytic Study of the Child*, 47, 1980, 159–187.

10 S. Freud, 'The psychogenesis of a case of homosexuality in a woman' [1920], *S. E.*, Vol. XVIII, pp. 145–175.

11 S. Freud, 'A case of paranoia running counter to the psychoanalytic theory of the disease' [1915], *S. E.*, Vol. XIV, pp. 261–273.

12 E. Young-Bruehl, *Anna Freud*, London, Macmillan, 1988.
13 Freud, 'Female sexuality' [1931] (see note 1); S. Freud, 'Femininity', Lecture XXXIII: *New Introductory Lectures on Psychoanalysis* [1933], *S. E.*, Vol. XXII, pp. 112–136.
14 Young-Bruehl, 1988 (see note 12).
15 S. Freud, 'A child is being beaten: A contribution to the study of the origin of sexual perversions' [1919], *S. E.*, Vol. XVII, pp. 175–205.
16 S. Freud, 'Some psychological consequences of the anatomical distinction between the sexes' [1925], *S. E.*, Vol. XIX, pp. 248–261.
17 P. Van Haute, 'Infantile sexuality, primary object-love and the anthropological significance of the Oedipus complex: Re-reading Freud's "Female sexuality" ', *International Journal of Psycho-Analysis*, 86, 2005, 1661–1678.
18 Freud, 'Femininity' [1933] (see note 13).
19 A. Freud, 'The relation of beating phantasies to a daydream', *International Journal of Psycho-Analysis* 4, 1923, 89–102; Young-Bruehl, 1988 (see note 12).
20 Freud 'Female sexuality' (see note 1).
21 Freud, 'Femininity' [1933] (see note 13).
22 R. S. Fisher, 'Lesbianism: Some developmental and psychodynamic consider-ations', *Psychoanalytic Inquiry*, 22, 2002, 278–295; D. Elisa, 'The primary maternal situation and female homoerotic desire', *Psychoanalytic Quarterly*, 22, 2002, 209–228.
23 J. Lampl-de Groot, 'The evolution of the Oedipus complex in women' [1927], in *The Development of the Mind*, New York, International Universities Press, 1965, pp. 3–19.
24 Freud, 'Femininity' [1933] (see note 13).
25 T. Laqueur, *Making Sex, Body and Gender from the Greeks to Freud*, Cambridge, MA, Harvard University Press, 1990.
26 Z. O. Fliegel, 'Women's development in analytic theory: Six decades of contro-versy', in J. L. Alpert (Ed.), *Psychoanalysis and Women: Contemporary Reappraisals*, Hillsdale, NJ, The Analytic Press, 1986, pp. 3–32.
27 M. Klein, 'The effects of early anxiety-situations on the sexual development of the girl', in *The Psycho-Analysis of Children* [1932], London, The Hogarth Press, 1973, pp. 268–325; R. Stoller, 'Primary femininity', *Journal of the American Psycho-Analytic Association, Supplement: Female Sexuality*, 24, 1976, 59–78; I. Fast, *Gender Identity, a Differentiation Model: Advances in Psychoanalysis: Theory, Research, and Practice*, Vol. 2, Hillsdale, NJ, The Analytic Press, 1984.
28 J. Chasseguet-Smirgel, 'Feminine guilt and the Oedipus complex' [1964], in J. Chasseguet-Smirgel (Ed.), *Female Sexuality*, London, Maresfield, 1970, pp. 94–134; J. Kestenberg, 'Outside and inside, male and female', *Journal of the American Psycho-Analytic Association* 16, 1968, 457–520; R. Edgecumbe, 'Some comments on the concepts of the negative oedipal phase in girls', *Psychoanalytic Study of the Child* 31, 1976, 35–62; M. V. Bergmann, 'The female Oedipus complex: Its antecedents and evolution', in Dale Mendell (Ed.), *Early Female Development, Current Psychoanalytic Views*, New York/London, SP Medical & Scientific Books, 1982, 61–80.
29 H. Roiphe & E. Galenson, *Infantile Origins of Sexual Identity*, New York, Inter-national Universities Press, 1981.
30 H. Parens, 'On the girl's psychosexual development: Reconsiderations suggested from direct observation', *Journal of the American Psycho-Analytic Association* 38, 1990, 743–772.
31 Edgecombe, 1976 (see note 28).
32 W. I. Grossman & W. A. Stewart, 'Penis envy: From childhood wish to

developmental metaphor', *Journal of the American Psycho-Analytic Association, Supplement: Female Sexuality*, 24, 1976, 193–212.

33 McDougall, 1995 (see note 2). A patient who was approaching 60 and, although she had been married, was never able to make love, told me that she used to wear men's underwear. She immediately recognized my question: whether she had never wanted to make the decision whether she was a man or a woman, because she would have preferred being both at the same time.

34 B. Grunberger, 'Outline for a study of narcissism in female sexuality' [1964], in J. Chasseguet-Smirgel, *Female Sexuality*, London, Maresfield, 1970, pp. 68–83.

35 L. Rotter, 'Zur Psychologie der weiblichen Sexualität', *Internationale Zeitschrift für Psychoanalyse* 20, 1934, 367–374.

36 M. Klein, 'Early stages of the Oedipus conflict and of super-ego formation' [1928], *The Psycho-Analysis of Children*, London, The Hogarth Press, 1973, pp. 179–209; J. Munder Ross, 'The eye of the beholder: The developmental dialogue between fathers and daughters', in Robert A. Nemiroff & Calvin A. Colarusso (Eds.), *New Dimensions in Adult Development*, New York, Basic Books, 1990, 47–72.

37 J. Benjamin, *Like Subjects, Love Objects: Essays on Recognition and Sexual Difference*, New Haven, CT, Yale University Press, 1995.

38 Chasseguet-Smirgel, 1964 (see note 28).

39 The transgenerational transmission of traumas is especially well known from the problematics of second-generation children of parent victims of the Second World War, but it is also more generally applicable: see, for example, A. Adelman, 'Traumatic memory and the intergenerational transmission of Holocaust narratives', *Psychoanalytic Study of the Child*, 50, 1995, 343–367; E. Kogan, *The Cry of Mute Children: A Psychoanalytic Perspective on the Second Generation of the Holocaust*, London/New York, Free Association Books, 1995.

40 W. W. Meissner, 'Gender identity and the self: II. Femininity, homosexuality, and the theory of the self', *Psychoanalytic Review*, 92, 2005, 29–66.

6 What does woman want?

1 E. K. Dahl, 'Daughters and mothers. Oedipal aspects of the witch-mother', *Psychoanalytic Study of the Child*, 44, 1989, 267–280; E. K. Dahl, 'Daughters and mothers. Aspects of the representational world during adolescence', *Psychoanalytic Study of the Child*, 50, 1995, 187–204.

2 R. L. Tyson & P. Tyson, *Psychoanalytic Theories of Development and Integration*, New Haven/London, Yale University Press, 1990.

3 N. Friday, *My Mother My Self*, London, Fontana Collins, 1977; N. Chodorow, *The Reproduction of Mothering: Psychoanalysis and the Sociology of Gender*, Berkeley, University of California Press, 1978.

4 Sophie Freud, *My Three Mothers and Other Passions*, New York/London, New York University Press, 1988.

5 J. Chasseguet-Smirgel, 'Feminine guilt and the Oedipus complex' [1964], in J. Chasseguet-Smirgel (Ed.), *Female Sexuality*, London, Maresfield, 1970, pp. 94–134.

6 M. M. Oliner, 'The anal phase', in Dale Mendell (Ed.), *Early Female Development: Current Psychoanalytic Views*, Lancaster, MTP Press, 1982, pp. 24–59.

7 D. K. Silverman, 'Female bonding: Some supportive findings for Melanie Klein's views', *Psychoanalytic Review* 74, 1987, 201–215.

8 D. Bernstein, *Female Identity Conflict in Clinical Practice*, Ed. N. Friedman & B. Distler, Northvale, NJ, Jason Aronson, 1993; R. L. Tyson & P. Tyson,

Psychoanalytic Theories of Development and Integration, New Haven/London, Yale University Press, 1990.

9 M. Torok, 'The significance of penis envy in women' [1964], in J. Chasseguet-Smirgel (Ed.), *Female Sexuality*, London, Maresfield, 1970, pp. 135–170.

10 K. Horney, 'On the genesis of the castration complex in women' [1924], in *Feminine Psychology*, New York, Norton, 1967, pp. 37–54.

11 H. E. Lerner, 'Parental mislabeling of female genitals as a determinant of penis envy and learning inhibitions in women', *Journal of the American Psycho-Analytic Association, Supplement: Female Psychology*, 24, 1976, 269–283.

12 H. Deutsch, *The Psychology of Women: A Psychoanalytic Interpretation*, Vol. I, New York, Grune & Stratton, 1944; H. Deutsch, *The Psychology of Women: A Psychoanalytic Interpretation*, Vol. II, New York, Grune & Stratton, 1945.

13 C. Sarnoff, *Latency*, New York, Jason Aronson, 1976.

14 M. Shopper, 'The rediscovery of the vagina and the importance of the menstrual tampon', in Max Sugar (Ed.), *Female Adolescent Development*, New York, Brunner/Mazel, 1979, pp. 214–233.

15 E. Young-Bruehl (Ed.), *Freud on Women*, New York/London, Norton & Company, 1990.

16 D. Pines, *A Woman's Unconscious Use of Her Body*, London, Virago, 1993.

17 A. Schwartz, 'Some notes on the development of female gender role identity', in J. L. Alpert (Ed.), *Psychoanalysis and Women: Contemporary Reappraisals*, Hillsdale, NJ, The Analytic Press, 1986, pp. 57–82.

18 S. Freud, 'A child is being beaten: A contribution to the study of the origin of sexual perversions' [1919], *S. E.*, Vol. XVII, pp. 175–205.

19 J. Benjamin, 'The alienation of desire: Women's masochism and ideal love', in J. L. Alpert (Ed.), *Psychoanalysis and Women: Contemporary Reappraisals*, Hillsdale, NJ, The Analytic Press, 1986, pp. 113–138; J. Benjamin, *The Bonds of Love: Psychoanalysis, Feminism and the Problem of Domination*, New York, Pantheon Books, 1988; J. Benjamin, *Like Subjects, Love Objects: Essays on Recognition and Sexual Difference*, New Haven, CT: Yale University Press, 1995.

20 E. Abelin, 'The role of the father in the separation–individuation process', in J. B. McDevitt & C. F. Settlage (Eds.), *Separation–Individuation*, New York, International Universities Press, 1971, pp. 229–252.

21 D. Holtzman & N. Kulish, 'The femininization of the female Oedipal complex: Part I: A reconsideration of the significance of separation issues', *Journal of the American Psycho-Analytic Association* 48, 2000, 1413–1437.

22 V. Woolf, *A Room of One's Own* [1928], Harmondsworth, UK, Penguin, 1970.

23 W. James, *The Varieties of Religious Experience* [1901–1902], New York, Doubleday, 1955.

7 Childbirth and depression

1 B. Pitt, 'Depression and childbirth', in E. S. Paykel (Ed.), *Handbook of Affective Disorders*, Edinburgh, Churchill Livingstone, 1982, pp. 361–378; I. F. Brockington, G. Winokur, & C. Dean, 'Puerperal psychosis', in I. F. Brockington & R. Kumar (Eds.), *Motherhood and Mental Illness*, London, Academic Press, 1982, pp. 37–69.

2 E. Esquirol, *Mental Maladies: A Treatise on Insanity*, Philadelphia, Lea & Blanchard, 1845; J. Conolly, 'Description and treatment of puerperal insanity', *Lancet*, 28 March 1846, 349–354.

3 D. W. Winnicott, 'Primary maternal preoccupation' [1956], *Collected Papers*, London, Tavistock, 1958, pp. 300–306.

4 S. Fraiberg, *Clinical Studies in Infant Mental Health: The First Year of Life*, New

York, Basic Books, 1980; E. J. Anthony, 'An overview of the effects of maternal depression on infant and child', in H. Morrison (Ed.), *Children of Depressed Parents: Risk, Identification and Intervention*, New York, Grune & Stratton, 1982.

5 H. Deutsch, *The Psychology of Women: A Psychoanalytic Interpretation*, Vol. I, New York, Grune & Stratton, 1944; H. Deutsch, *The Psychology of Women: A Psychoanalytic Interpretation*, Vol. II, New York, Grune & Stratton, 1945.

6 Anna Freud, *The Ego and the Mechanisms of Defence* [1936], New York, International Universities Press, 1966.

7 S. Freud, 'Femininity', Lecture XXXIII. *New Introductory Lectures on Psychoanalysis* [1933], *S. E.*, Vol. XXII, pp. 112–136.

8 D. W. Winnicott, 'The relationship of a mother to her baby at the beginning', *The Family and Individual Development*, London, Tavistock, 1965, pp. 15–20.

8 Martha: A woman in her middle years

1 E. Jacques, 'The midlife crisis', in S. I. Greenspan & G. H. Pollock (Eds.), *The Course of Life: Psychoanalytic Contributions towards Understanding Personality Development*, Vol. III, *Adulthood and the Aging Process*, Adelphi, MD, Mental Health Study Center, 1981, pp. 1–23; D. L. Gutmann 'Psychoanalysis and aging. A developmental view', in S. I. Greenspan & G. H. Pollock (Eds.), *The Course of Life: Psychoanalytic Contributions towards Understanding Personality Development*, Vol. III, *Adulthood and the Aging Process*, Adelphi, MD, Mental Health Study Center, 1981, pp. 81–100.

2 Erik Erikson, 'Themes of adulthood in the Freud–Jung correspondence', in Neil J. Smelser & Erik H. Erikson (Eds.), *Themes of Love and Work in Adulthood*, Cambridge, MA, Harvard University Press, 1980, pp. 43–77.

3 R. Formanek, 'Learning the lines: Women's aging and self-esteem', in J. L. Alpert (Ed.), *Psychoanalysis and Women: Contemporary Reappraisals*, Hillsdale, NJ, The Analytic Press, 1986, pp. 139–160.

4 D. L., Gutmann, 'Psychological development and pathology in later adulthood', in Robert A. Nemiroff & Calvin A. Colarusso (Eds.), *New Dimensions in Adult Development*, New York, Basic Books, 1990, 170–185.

5 H. Meyers, 'The impact of teenage children on parents', in J. M. Oldham & R. S. Liebert (Eds.), *The Middle Years: New Psychoanalytic Perspectives*, New Haven/London, Yale University Press, 1989, pp. 75–88.

6 Others mention middle age as the third separation–individuation phase (see also note 15).

7 L. Rubin, *Women of a Certain Age: The Midlife Search for Self*, New York, Harper & Row, 1979; G. H. Pollock, 'Aging or aged: Development or pathology', in S. I. Greenspan & G. H. Pollock (Eds.), *The Course of Life: Psychoanalytic Contributions towards Understanding Personality Development*, Vol. III, *Adulthood and the Aging Process*, Adelphi, MD, Mental Health Study Center, 1981; O. Kernberg, 'Normal narcissism in middle age, and pathological narcissism in middle age', *Internal World and External Reality Object Relations Theory Applied*, New York/London, Jason Aronson, 1980, pp. 121–134, 135–154; O. Kernberg, 'The interaction of middle age and character pathology', in J. M. Oldham & R. S. Liebert (Eds.), *The Middle Years: New Psychoanalytic Perspectives*, New Haven/London, Yale University Press, 1989, pp. 209–223; E. L. Auchincloss & R. Michels, 'The impact of middle age on ambitions and ideals', in Oldham & Liebert, 1989, pp. 40–75; M. Kirkpatrick, 'Lesbians: A different middle age', in Oldham & Liebert, 1989, pp. 135–148; A. H. Modell, 'Object relations theory: Psychic aliveness in the middle years', in Oldham & Liebert, 1989, pp. 17–26;

J. Oldham, 'The third individuation: Middle aged children and their parents', in Oldham & Liebert, 1989, pp. 89–104; P. Ornstein, 'Self psychology: The fate of the nuclear self in the middle years', in Oldham & Liebert, 1989, pp. 27–39; G. E. Vaillant, 'The evolution of defense mechanisms during the middle years', in Oldham & Liebert, 1989, pp. 58–72; M. Viederman, 'Middle life as a period of mutative change', in Oldham & Liebert, 1989, pp. 224–239; G. Greer, *The Change: Women, Aging and the Menopause*, London, Hamish Hamilton, 1991; G. Sheehy, *Silent Passages*, Houston/New York, Random House, 1976.

8 S. Freud, 'The disposition to obsessional neurosis' [1913], *S. E.*, Vol. XII, pp. 317–327.

9 S. Freud, 'Femininity', Lecture XXXIII. New Introductory Lectures on Psycho-analysis [1933], *S. E.*, Vol. XXII, pp. 112–136.

10 T. Benedek, 'Climacterium: A developmental phase', *Psychoanalytic Quarterly* 19, 1950, 1–27.

11 H. S. Kaplan, 'Sex, intimacy and the aging process', *Journal of the American Academy of Psychoanalysis* 18, 1990, 185–205.

12 H. P Hildebrand, 'The other side of the wall: A psychoanalytic study of creativity in later life', in R. A. Nemiroff, & C. A. Colarusso (Eds.), *New Dimensions in Adult Development*, New York, Basic Books, 1990, pp. 467–486.

13 Gutmann, 1990 (see note 4).

14 Meyers, 1989 (see note 5); Oldham & Liebert, 1989 (see note 5); C. A. Colarusso & R. A. Nemiroff, *Adult Development: A New Dimension in Psychodynamic Theory and Practice*, New York/London, Plenum Press, 1981.

15 S. Freud, 'Female sexuality' [1931], *S. E.*, Vol. XXI, pp. 223–243.

16 W. R. Bion, *Attention and Interpretation*, London, Maresfield, 1970.

17 I. Freud, *Mannen en moeders. De levenslange worsteling van zonen met hun moeders* [Men and mothers. The lifelong struggle of sons and their mothers], Amsterdam, Van Gennep, 2002.

18 P. King, 'The life cycle as indicated by the nature of the transference in the psycho-analysis of the middle aged and elderly', *International Journal of Psycho-Analysis* 61, 1980, 153–160.

19 M. Klein, 'A contribution to the psychogenesis of manic-depressive states' [1935], in *Love, Guilt and Reparation, and Other Works (1921–1945)*, London, The Hogarth Press, 1975, 262–289.

20 E. Young-Bruehl, 'Looking for Anna Freud's mother', *Psychoanalytic Study of the Child* 44, 1989, 391–408.

21 See Erikson, 1980 (see note 2).

9 On rejected mothers

1 Hella de Jonge, *Los van de wereld* [Detached from the world], Amsterdam, Balans, 2006.

2 Irène Némirovski, *Suite Francaise*, tr. Sandra Smith, New York, Knopf, 2006.

3 Pearl King & Riccardo Steiner (Eds.), *The Freud–Klein Controversies 1941–45*, London, New Library of Psychoanalysis, Tavistock, 1991.

4 Nicholas Wright, *Mrs. Klein*, London, Walker Books, 1988.

10 History and hysteria

1 S. Freud & J. Breuer, *Studies on Hysteria* [1895], *S. E.*, Vol. II, 1–153.

2 DSM–IV, *Diagnostic and Statistical Manual of Mental Disorders*, 4th ed., Washington, DC, American Psychiatric Association, 1994.

3 Freud [1905] (ch 5, note 8).

4 I. Veith, *The History of Disease*, Chicago, The University of Chicago Press, 1965.

5 Freud & Breuer [1895] (see note 1).

6 O. Kernberg, *Borderline Conditions and Pathological Narcissism*, New York, Jason Aronson, 1975; O. Kernberg, *Object Relations Theory and Clinical Psychoanalysis*, New York, Jason Aronson, 1976.

7 A. Krohn, *Hysteria, the Elusive Neurosis*, New York, International Universities Press, 1978; S. Mentzos, *Hysterie. Zur Psychodynamik unbewuszter Inszenierungen*, Frankfurt am Main, Fischer, 1993; M. J. Horowitz (Ed.), *Hysterical Personality*, New York, Jason Aronson, 1977; M. J. Horowitz (Ed.), *Hysterical Personality Style and the Histrionic Personality Disorder*, Northvale, NJ/London, Jason Aronson, 1991.

8 J. M. Charcot, *Leçons sur les maladies du système nerveux*, Vol. 3, Paris, 1886; Charcot, 1886, translated into German by S. Freud, *Neue Vorlesungen über die Krankheiten des Nervensystems, insbesondere über Hysterie*, Leipzig/Vienna, Toeplitz & Deuticke, 1886.

9 H. F. Ellenberger, *The Discovery of the Unconscious: The History and Evolution of Dynamic Psychiatry*, New York, Basic Books, 1970; P. Gay, *Freud: A Life for Our Time*, London/Melbourne, J. M. Dent & Sons, 1988; G. Gödde, 'Charcots neurologische Hysterietheorie. Vom Aufstieg und Niedergang eines wissenschaftlichen Paradigmas', *Lucifer-Amor, Zeitschrift zur Geschichte der Pschoanalyse. Geschichte der Hysterie* 7, 1994, 7–51.

10 S. Freud, 'Further remarks on the neuro-psychoses of defence' [1896], *S. E.*, Vol. III, pp. 159–189.

11 W. James, *The Principles of Psychology*, Vol. I [1890], New York, Dover Publications, 1950; Ellenberger, 1970 (see note 8).

12 H. S. Decker, *Freud, Dora, and Vienna 1900*, New York, The Free Press, 1991.

13 A. Hirschmüller, *The Life and Work of Josef Breuer*, New York/London, New York University Press, 1989.

14 Freud & Breuer [1895] (see note 1).

15 Freud [1905] (ch 5, note 8).

16 J. Kerr, *A Most Dangerous Method: The Story of Jung, Freud and Sabina Spielrein*, London, Sinclair-Stevenson, 1994; H. C. Halberstadt-Freud, 'De vrouwengek in de psychoanalyse' [The ladies' man in psychoanalysis], *NCR Handelsblad*, 23 April 1994, Weekly book section.

17 Freud & Breuer [1895] (see note 1).

18 M. Krüll, *Freud und sein Vater. Die Entstehung der Psychoanalyse und Freuds ungelöste Vaterbindung*, Munich, Verlag C. H. Beck, 1979.

19 Before rejecting what Kris later called the 'seduction theory', Freud had held several trauma theories in rapid succession. E. Kris, *The Origins of Psychoanalysis*, New York, Basic Books, 1954; R. B. Blass & B. Simon, 'Freud on his own mistakes: The role of seduction in the etiology of neurosis', J. H. Smith & H. Morris (Eds.), *Telling Facts: History and Narration in Psychoanalysis*, Baltimore/London, Johns Hopkins University Press, 1992, pp. 161–183; R. B. Blass & B. Simon, 'The value of the historical perspective to contemporary psychoanalysis: Freud's "seduction hypothesis"', *International Journal of Psycho-Analysis* 75, 1994, 677–694.

20 S. Freud, Letter of May 1897, in J. M. Masson (Ed.), *The Complete Letters of Sigmund Freud to Wilhelm Fliess, 1887–1904*, Cambridge, MA/London, The Belknap Press of Harvard University Press, 1985.

21 Revisionists such as Jeffrey M. Masson, and later Alice Miller and the Dutch Han Israëls, are just as wrong and equally reductionist and biased as are the

psychoanalysts who adhere to the opinion that Freud suddenly rejected his so-called seduction theory. The former claim that he did so in a calculated manner, the latter that it occurred strictly on the basis of the discovery of the Oedipus complex. The historical state inside Freud's head is more complicated, however, more subtle and gradual, as the Israeli psychologist Rachel Blass and the American psychologist Bennette Simon have explained in various articles – a fascinating account of their common research. They show how Freud struggled with his own desires and projections and their interaction with his scientific arguments.

22 B. Simon, 'Is the Oedipus complex still the cornerstone of psychoanalysis?', *Journal of the American Psycho-Analytic Association* 39, 1991, 641–668; B. Simon & R. Blass, 'Developments and vicissitudes of Freud's ideas on the Oedipus complex', in J. Neu (Ed.), *The Cambridge Companion to Freud*, Cambridge, Cambridge University Press, 1991, pp. 161–174.

23 I. Freud, *Mannen en moeders. De levenslange worsteling van zonen met hun moeders* [Men and mothers. The lifelong struggle of sons and their mothers], Amsterdam, Van Gennep, 2002.

24 This work was later continued by others: K. H. Blacker & J. P. Turpin, 'Hysteria and hysterical structures: Developmental and social theories', in M. J. Horowitz (Ed.), *Hysterical Personality*, New York, Jason Aronson, 1977, pp. 95–142; see also M. J. Horowitz (Ed.), *Hysterical Personality Style and the Histrionic Personality*, Northvale, NJ/London, Jason Aronson, 1991, pp. 15–66.

25 J. S. Grotstein, 'Reflections on a century of Freud: Some paths not chosen', *British Journal of Psychotherapy* 9, 1992, pp. 181–187; W. R. D. Fairbairn, 'Observations on the nature of hysteria', *Journal of Medical Psychology* 27, 1954, 105–125; I. Brenner, 'The dissociative character: A reconsideration of "multiple personality" ', *Journal of the American Psycho-Analytic Association* 42, 1994, 819–846.

26 W. Stekel, *Nervöse Angstzustände und ihre Behandlung*, Berlin/Vienna, Verlag Urban & Schwarzenberg, 1908 (first German ed., with a Foreword by Sigmund Freud).

27 O. Fenichel, *The Psychoanalytic Theory of Neurosis*, London, Routledge & Kegan Paul, 1946.

28 W. Reich, *Character Analysis* [1948], New York, The Noonday Press, Farrar, Straus & Cudahy, 1961.

29 L. Rangell, 'The nature of conversion', *Journal of the American Psycho-Analytic Association* 7, 1959, 632–662; J. O. Wisdom, 'A methodological approach to the problem of hysteria', *International Journal of Psycho-Analysis* 42, 1961, 224–237.

30 Zetzel, E. 'Contribution to a symposium on indications and contra-indications for psychoanalytic treatment: The so-called good hysteric', *International Journal of Psycho-Analysis* 49, 1968, 256–260.

31 E. Brenman, 'Hysteria', *International Journal of Psycho-Analysis* 66, 1985, 423–432.

32 S. L. Gilman, H. King, R. Porter, G. S. Rousseau, & E. Schowalter, *Hysteria beyond Freud*, Los Angeles/London, University of California Press, 1993.

33 E. de Wind, 'Some implications of former massive traumatization upon the actual analytic process', *International Journal of Psycho-Analysis* 65, 1984, 273–281.

34 B. Simon, ' "Incest – see under Oedipus complex". The history of an error in psychoanalysis', *Journal of the American Psycho-Analytic Association* 40, 1992, 955–988.

35 Storr, A. 'The myth of repressed memory: False memories and allegations of sexual abuse', *International Herald Tribune*, 23 January 1995, 7.

36 E. F. Loftus, 'The reality of repressed memories', *American Psychologist* 48, 1993, 518–537.

37 F. Crews, 'The unknown Freud', *New York Review of Books*, 18 November 1993, 61–66. See also the discussions in the *New York Review of Books*, 3 February 1994, 34–43; 1 December 1994, 49–57; 12 January 1995, 42–47.

38 A. Miller, *Du sollst nicht merken*, Frankfurt am Main, Suhrkamp, 1981.

39 J. M. Masson, *The Assault on Truth: Freud's Suppression of the Seduction Theory*, New York, Farrar, Straus & Giroux, 1984.

40 Brenman, 1985 (see note 30).

41 S. Freud, 'Hysterical phantasies and their relation to bisexuality' [1908], *S.E.*, Vol. IX, 155–167; S. Freud, 'Some general remarks on hysterical attacks' [1909], *S.E.*, Vol. IX, 227–235.

42 D. Shapiro, *Neurotic Styles*, New York, Basic Books, 1965; E. Shorter, *From Paralysis to Fatigue: A History of Psychosomatic Illness in the Modern Era*, New York, Simon & Schuster, 1992; E. Showalter, *Hystories: Hysterical Epidemics and Modern Culture*, New York/London, Columbia University Press/Picador, 1997.

43 R. Wagner, *Siegfried*, Stuttgart, Reclam, 1995.

44 S. van het Hof, *Anorexia Nervosa, The Historical and Cultural Specificity: Fallacious Theories and Tenacious Facts*, Lisse, Swets & Zeitlinger, 1994.

Bibliography

Abelin, E. (1971). 'The role of the father in the separation–individuation process', in J. B. McDevitt & C. F. Settlage (Eds.), *Separation–Individuation*. New York, International Universities Press, pp. 229–252.

Adelman, A. (1995). Traumatic memory and the intergenerational transmission of Holocaust narratives'. *Psychoanalytic Study of the Child*, 50, 343–367.

Aeschylus (1977). *Oresteia: Agamemnon*, tr. Robert Fagles. Harmondsworth, UK, Penguin.

Alpert, J. L. (Ed.) (1986). *Psychoanalysis and Women: Contemporary Reappraisals*. Hillsdale, NJ, The Analytic Press.

Anthony, E. J. (1982). 'An overview of the effects of maternal depression on infant and child', in H. Morrison (Ed.), *Children of Depressed Parents: Risk, Identification and Intervention*. New York, Grune & Stratton, pp. 1–16.

Ariès, P. (1973). *L'enfant et la vie familiale sous l'ancien régime*. Paris, Seuil.

Ariès, P. (1979) 'Entretien'. *Nouvelle Revue de Psychanalyse, L'enfant*, 19, 13–26.

Auchincloss, E. L., & Michels, R. (1989). 'The impact of middle age on ambitions and ideals', in J. Oldham & R. S. Liebert (Eds.), *The Middle Years*. New Haven, Yale University Press, pp. 40–75.

Augustine of Hippo (1961). *Confessions*. Harmondsworth, UK, Penguin Classics.

Badinter, E. (1980). *L'amour en plus. Histoire de l'amour maternel (XVIIe–XXe siècle)*. Paris, Flammarion.

Balsam, R. H. (2000). 'The mother within the mother'. *Psychoanalytic Quarterly*, 69, 465–492.

Benedek, T. (1950). 'Climacterium: A developmental phase'. *Psychoanalytic Quarterly* 19, 1–27.

Benjamin, J. (1986). 'The alienation of desire: Women's masochism and ideal love', in J. L. Alpert (Ed.), *Psychoanalysis and Women: Contemporary Reappraisals*. Hillsdale, NJ, The Analytic Press, pp. 113–138.

Benjamin, J. (1988). *The Bonds of Love: Psychoanalysis, Feminism and the Problem of Domination*. New York, Pantheon Books.

Benjamin, J. (1995). *Like Subjects, Love Objects: Essays on Recognition and Sexual Difference*. New Haven, Yale University Press.

Bergmann, M. V. (1982). 'The female Oedipus complex: Its antecedents and evolution', in Dale Mendell (Ed.), *Early Female Development, Current Psychoanalytic Views*. New York/London, SP Medical & Scientific Books, 61–80.

Bernstein, B. P. (2004). 'Mothers and daughters from today's psychoanalytic perspective'. *Psychoanalytic Inquiry*, 24, 601–628.

Bernstein, D. (1993). *Female Identity Conflict in Clinical Practice*, Ed. N. Friedman & B. Distler. Northvale, NJ, Jason Aronson.

Bion, W. R. (1970). *Attention and Interpretation*. London, Maresfield.

Blacker, K. H. & Turpin, J. P. (1977). 'Hysteria and hysterical structures: Developmental and social theories', in M. J. Horowitz (Ed.), *Hysterical Personality*. New York, Jason Aronson, pp. 95–142.

Blass, R. B. (1980). 'Did Dora have an Oedipus complex? A re-examination of the theoretical context of Freud's "Fragments of an analysis" '. *Psychoanalytic Study of the Child*, 47, 159–187.

Blass, R. & Simon, B. (1992). 'Freud on his own mistakes: The role of seduction in the etiology of neurosis', in J. H. Smith & H. Morris (Eds.), *Telling Facts: History and Narration in Psychoanalysis*. Baltimore/London, Johns Hopkins University Press, pp. 161–183.

Blass, R. & Simon, B. (1994). 'The value of the historical perspective to contemporary psychoanalysis: Freud's "seduction hypothesis" '. *International Journal of Psycho-Analysis* 75, 677–694.

Blos, P. (1967). 'The second individuation process of adolescence'. *Psychoanalytic Study of the Child*, 22, 162–187.

Blos, P. (1985). *Son and Father*. London, The Free Press.

Blum, H. P. (1981). 'The maternal ego-ideal and the regulation of maternal qualities', in G. H. Pollock & S. I. Greenspan (Eds.), *The Course of Life, Psychoanalytic Contributions towards Understanding Personality Development*, Vol. III, *Adulthood and the Aging Process*. Adelphi, MA, Mental Health Study Center, pp. 91–114.

Boswell, J. (1990). *The Kindness of Strangers: The Abandonment of Children in Western Europe from Late Antiquity to the Renaissance*. New York, Vintage Books.

Bowlby, J. (1951). *Maternal Care and Mental Health*. Geneva, World Health Organization.

Brazelton, T. B. & Cramer, B. (1991). *The Earliest Relationship: Parents, Infants and the Drama of Early Attachment*. London, Karnac Books.

Brenman, E. (1985). 'Hysteria'. *International Journal of Psycho-Analysis* 66, 423–432.

Brenner, I. (1994). 'The dissociative character: A reconsideration of "multiple personality" '. *Journal of the American Psycho-Analytic Association* 42, 819–846.

Brockington, I. F., & Kumar, R. (Eds.) (1982). *Motherhood and Mental Illness*. London, Academic Press.

Catalogue North-Brabants Museum (1997). *Kinderen van alle tijden*. Zwolle, Waanders, 'sHertogenbosch.

Charcot, J. M. (1886). *Leçons sur les maladies du système nerveux*, Vol. 3. Paris.

Chasseguet-Smirgel, J. (Ed.) (1970). *Female Sexuality*. London, Maresfield.

Chodorow, N. (1978). *The Reproduction of Mothering: Psychoanalysis and the Sociology of Gender*. Berkeley, University of California Press.

Chodorow, N. (1992). 'Heterosexuality as a compromise formation: Reflections on the psycho-analytic theory of sexual development'. *Psychoanalysis and Contemporary Thought*, 15, 267–302.

Chodorow, N. (1994). *Femininities, Masculinities, Sexualities: Freud and Beyond*. London, Free Association Books.

Colarusso, C. A. & Nemiroff, R. A. (1981). *Adult Development: A New Dimension in Psychodynamic Theory and Practice*. New York/London, Plenum Press.

Conolly, J. (1846). 'Description and treatment of puerperal insanity'. *Lancet*, 28 March, 349–354.

Crews, F. (1993). 'The unknown Freud'. *New York Review of Books*, 18 November, 61–66.

Cunningham, H. (1995). *Children and Childhood in Western Society since 1500*. London/New York, Longman.

Dahl, E. K. (1989). 'Daughters and mothers: Oedipal aspects of the witch-mother'. *Psychoanalytic Study of the Child*, 44, 267–280.

Dahl, E. K. (1995). 'Daughters and mothers: Aspects of the representational world during adolescence'. *Psychoanalytic Study of the Child*, 50, 187–204.

Dally, A. (1982). *Inventing Motherhood: The Consequences of an Ideal*. London, Burnett.

Decker, H. S. (1991). *Freud, Dora, and Vienna 1900*. New York, The Free Press.

deMause, L. (Ed.) (1974). *The History of Childhood*. New York, Harper.

Dervin, D. (1998). 'The Electra complex: A history of misrepresentations'. *Gender and Psychoanalysis* 4, 451–470.

Deutsch, H. (1944). *The Psychology of Women: A Psychoanalytic Interpretation*, Vol. I. New York, Grune & Stratton.

Deutsch, H. (1945). *The Psychology of Women: A Psychoanalytic Interpretation*, Vol. II. New York, Grune & Stratton.

Donzelot, J. (1977). *La police des familles*. Paris, Editions de Minuit.

DSM–IV (1994). *Diagnostic and Statistical Manual of Mental Disorders*, 4th ed. Washington, DC, American Psychiatric Association.

Edgecumbe, R. (1976). 'Some comments on the concepts of the negative Oedipal phase in girls'. *Psychoanalytic Study of the Child* 31, 35–62.

Elias, N. (1994). *The Civilizing Process: Sociogenetic and Psychogenetic Investigations*, rev. ed. Oxford, Blackwell.

Elisa, D. (2002). 'The primary maternal situation and female homoerotic desire'. *Psychoanalytic Quarterly*, 22, 209–228.

Ellenberger, H. F. (1970). *The Discovery of the Unconscious: The History and Evolution of Dynamic Psychiatry*. New York, Basic Books.

Erikson, E. (1980). 'Themes of adulthood in the Freud–Jung correspondence', in N. J. Smelser & E. H. Erikson (Eds.), *Themes of Love and Work in Adulthood*. Cambridge, MA, Harvard University Press, pp. 43–77.

Esquirol, E. (1845). *Mental Maladies: A Treatise on Insanity*. Philadelphia, Lea & Blanchard.

Euripides (1999). *Electra and other Plays*, tr. R. Rutherford & J. Davie. Harmondsworth, UK, Penguin.

Fairbairn, W. R. D. (1954). 'Observations on the nature of hysteria'. *Journal of Medical Psychology* 27, 105–125.

Fast, I. (1984). *Gender Identity, a Differentiation Model: Advances in Psychoanalysis: Theory, Research, and Practice*, Vol. 2. Hillsdale, NJ, The Analytic Press.

Fenichel, O. (1946). *The Psychoanalytic Theory of Neurosis*. London, Routledge & Kegan Paul.

Fisher, R. S. (2002). 'Lesbianism: Some developmental and psychodynamic considerations'. *Psychoanalytic Inquiry*, 22, 278–295.

Fliegel, Z. O. (1986). 'Women's development in analytic theory: Six decades of controversy', in J. L. Alpert (Ed.), *Psychoanalysis and Women: Contemporary Reappraisals*. Hillsdale, NJ, The Analytic Press, pp. 3–32.

Fonagy, P., & Target, M. (1996). 'Playing with reality I: Theory of mind and the normal development of psychic reality'. *International Journal of Psycho-Analysis*, 77, 2, 217–235.

Formanek, R. (1986). 'Learning the lines: Women's aging and self-esteem', in J. L. Alpert (Ed.), *Psychoanalysis and Women: Contemporary Reappraisals*. Hillsdale, NJ, The Analytic Press, pp. 139–160.

Foucault, M. (1961). *Histoire de la folie*. Paris, Plon.

Fraiberg, S. (1980). *Clinical Studies in Infant Mental Health: The First Year of Life*. New York, Basic Books.

Freud, A. (1966 [1936]). *The Ego and the Mechanisms of Defense*. New York, International Universities Press.

Freud, A. (1973). *Infants without Families: Report on the Hampstead Nurseries 1939–1945*. New York, International Universities Press.

Freud, I. (2002). *Mannen en moeders. De levenslange worsteling van zonen met hun moeders* [Men and mothers. The lifelong struggle of sons and their mothers]. Amsterdam, Van Gennep.

Freud, S. (1886). *Neue Vorlesungen über die Krankheiten des Nervensystems, insbesondere über Hysterie*. Leipzig/Vienna, Toeplitz & Deuticke.

Freud, S. (1971). *The Standard Edition of the Complete Psychological Works of Sigmund Freud*. London, The Hogarth Press.

Freud, S. & Breuer, J. (1895), *Studien über Hysterie*. Leipzig/Vienna, Deuticke.

Freud, Sophie (1988). *My Three Mothers and Other Passions*. New York/London, New York University Press.

Friday, N. (1977). *My Mother My Self*. London, Fontana Collins.

Frijhoff, W. (1984). 'Impasses en beloften van de mentaliteitsgeschiedenis'. *Tijdschrift voor Sociale Geschiedenis* 10, 406–437.

Gay, P. (1988). *Freud: A Life for Our Time*. London/Melbourne, J. M. Dent & Sons.

Gilman, S. L., King, H., Porter, R., Rousseau, G. S., & Schowalter, E. (1993). *Hysteria beyond Freud*. Los Angeles/London, University of California Press.

Giraudoux, J. (1937). *Electre*. Paris, Grasset.

Gödde, G. (1994). 'Charcots neurologische Hysterietheorie. Vom Aufstieg und Niedergang eines wissenschaftlichen Paradigmas'. *Lucifer-Amor, Zeitschrift zur Geschichte der Pschoanalyse. Geschichte der Hysterie* 7, 7–51.

Greer, G. (1991). *The Change: Women, Aging and the Menopause*. London, Hamish Hamilton.

Grimal, P. (1986). *Dictionary of Classical Mythology*. Oxford/New York, Blackwell.

Grossman, W. I., & Stewart, W. A. (1976). 'Penis envy: From childhood wish to developmental metaphor'. *Journal of the American Psycho-Analytic Association, Supplement: Female Sexuality*, 24, 193–212.

Grotstein, J. S. (1992). 'Reflections on a century of Freud: Some paths not chosen'. *British Journal of Psychotherapy* 9, 181–187.

Grunberger, B. (1970 [1964]). 'Outline for a study of narcissism in female sexuality', in J. Chasseguet-Smirgel, *Female Sexuality*. London, Maresfield, pp. 68–83.

Gutmann, D. L. (1980). 'Psychoanalysis and aging: A developmental view', in S. I. Greenspan & G. H. Pollock (Eds.), *The Course of Life: Psychoanalytic*

Contributions towards Understanding Personality Development, Vol. III, *Adulthood and the Aging Process*. Adelphi, MD, Mental Health Study Center, pp. 81–100.

Gutmann, D. L. (1990). 'Psychological development and pathology in later adulthood', in Robert A. Nemiroff & Calvin A. Colarusso (Eds.), *New Dimensions in Adult Development*. New York, Basic Books, pp. 170–185.

Haks, D. (1982). *Huwelijk en gezin in Holland in de 17e en 18e eeuw* [Marriage and family in Holland in the seventeenth and eighteenth centuries]. Assen, Van Gorcum.

Halberstadt-Freud, H. C. (1994). 'Patient, colleague, mistress on an exploration of the Freud–Jung–Sabina Spielrein triangle', *European Élan, Culture, Life & Style*, 11–17 March 1994, No. 200. [Book review of Kerr, J. (1994) *A most dangerous method: The story of Jung, Freud and Sabina Spielrein*. London: Sinclair Stevenson].

Halberstadt-Freud, H. C. (1995). 'Clara Schumann: "A woman's love and life: A psychoanalytic interpretation" '. *The Psychohistory Review*, 23, 2, Winter, 143–166.

Halberstadt-Freud, H.C. (1994). 'Patient, colleague, mistress on an exploration of the Freud-Jung-Sabina Spielrein triangle', *European Élan, Culture, Life & Style*, 11–17 March 1994, No. 200. [Book review of Kerr, J. (1994) *A most dangerous method: The story of Jung, Freud and Sabina Spielrein*. London: Sinclair Stevenson].

Harris, B. (1979). 'Two lives, one 24-hour day', in A. Roland & B. Harris (Eds.), *Career and Motherhood: Struggles for a New Identity*. New York, Human Sciences Press, pp. 24–45.

Héroard, J. (1979). 'Extraits du Journal d'Héroard (1601–1628) sur l'enfance et la jeunesse de Louis XIII'. *Nouvelle Revue de Psychanalyse* 19, 268–330.

Hildebrand, H. P. (1990). 'The other side of the wall: A psychoanalytic study of creativity in later life', in R. A. Nemiroff, & C. A. Colarusso (Eds.), *New Dimensions in Adult Development*. New York, Basic Books, pp. 467–486.

Hirschmüller, A. (1989). *The Life and Work of Josef Breuer*. New York/London, New York University Press.

Hof, S. van het (1994). *Anorexia Nervosa, the Historical and Cultural Specificity: Fallacious Theories and Tenacious Facts*, Lisse, Swets & Zeitlinger.

Hofmannsthal, H. von (1908). *Electra*. London, Boosey & Hawkes.

Holtzman, D. & Kulish, N. (2000). 'The femininization of the female Oedipal complex: Part I: A reconsideration of the significance of separation issues'. *Journal of the American Psycho-Analytic Association* 48, 1413–1437.

Horney, K. (1967) *Feminine Psychology*. New York, Norton.

Horowitz, M. J. (Ed.) (1977). *Hysterical Personality*. New York, Jason Aronson.

Horowitz, M. J. (Ed.) (1991). *Hysterical Personality Style and the Histrionic Personality Disorder*. Northvale, NJ/London, Jason Aronson.

Huizinga, J. (1999). *Herfsttij der middeleeuwen* [Autumn of the Middle Ages]. Amsterdam, Contact.

Halberstadt, H. C. (1994). 'De vrouwengek in de psychoanalyse' [The ladies' man in psychoanalysis]. *NCR Handelsblad*, 23 April, Weekly book section.

Jacques, E. (1981). 'The midlife crisis', in S. I. Greenspan & G. H. Pollock (Eds.), *The Course of Life: Psychoanalytic Contributions towards Understanding Personality Development*, Vol. III, *Adulthood and the Aging Process*. Adelphi, MD, Mental Health Study Center, pp. 1–23.

James, W. (1950 [1890]). *The Principles of Psychology*, Vol. I. New York, Dover Publications.

James, W. (1955 [1901–1902]). *The Varieties of Religious Experience*. New York, Doubleday.

Jonge, Hella de (2006). *Los van de wereld* [Detached from the world]. Amsterdam, Balans.

Jung, C. G. (1971). *Freud und die Psychoanalyse. Versuch einer Darstellung der psychoanalytischen Theorie. Gesammelte Werke, Vol. 4*. Olten, Walter Verlag.

Kaplan, H. S. (1990). 'Sex, intimacy and the aging process'. *Journal of the American Academy of Psychoanalysis* 18, 185–205.

Kaplan, L. J. (1991). *Female Perversions*. London, Pandora Press.

Kernberg, O. (1975). *Borderline Conditions and Pathological Narcissism*. New York, Jason Aronson.

Kernberg, O. (1976). *Object Relations Theory and Clinical Psychoanalysis*. New York, Jason Aronson.

Kernberg, O. (1980). *Internal World and External Reality: Object Relations Theory Applied*. New York/London, Jason Aronson.

Kernberg, O. (1989). 'The interaction of middle age and character pathology', in J. M. Oldham & R. S. Liebert (Eds.), *The Middle Years: New Psychoanalytic Perspectives*. New Haven/London, Yale University Press, pp. 209–223.

Kerr, J. (1994). *A Most Dangerous Method: The Story of Jung, Freud and Sabina Spielrein*. London, Sinclair-Stevenson.

Kestenberg, J. (1968). 'Outside and inside, male and female'. *Journal of the American Psycho-Analytic Association* 16, 457–520.

Khan, M. M. (1979). 'The role of polymorph-perverse body experiences and object-relations in ego-integration' [1962], in C. Yorke (Ed.), *Alienation in Perversions*. London, The Hogarth Press, pp. 31–55.

King, P. (1980). 'The life cycle as indicated by the nature of the transference in the psychoanalysis of the middle aged and elderly'. *International Journal of Psycho-Analysis* 61, 153–160.

King, P. & Steiner, R. (Eds.) (1991). *The Freud–Klein Controversies 1941–45*. London, New Library of Psychoanalysis, Tavistock.

Kirkpatrick, M. (1989). 'Lesbians: A different middle age', in J. M. Oldham & R. S. Liebert (Eds.), *The Middle Years: New Psychoanalytic Perspectives*. New Haven/London, Yale University Press, pp. 135–148.

Klein, M. (1975). *Love, Guilt and Reparation, and Other Works (1921–1945)*. London, The Hogarth Press.

Klein, M. (1973). *The Psycho-Analysis of Children*. London, The Hogarth Press.

Kogan, E. (1995). *The Cry of Mute Children: A Psychoanalytic Perspective on the Second Generation of the Holocaust*. London/New York, Free Association Books.

Kris, E. (1954). *The Origins of Psychoanalysis*. New York, Basic Books.

Krohn, A. (1978). *Hysteria, the Elusive Neurosis*. New York, International Universities Press.

Krüll, M. (1979). *Freud und sein Vater. Die Entstehung der Psychoanalyse und Freuds ungelöste Vaterbindung*. Munich, Verlag C. H. Beck.

Lampl-de Groot, J. (1965 [1927]). 'The evolution of the Oedipus complex in women', in J. Lampl-de Groot, *The Development of the Mind*. New York, International Universities Press, pp. 3–19.

Laqueur, T. (1990). *Making Sex, Body and Gender from the Greeks to Freud*. Cambridge, MA, Harvard University Press.

Laslett, P. (1965). *The World We Have Lost*. London, Methuen.

Laslett, P. (1977). *Family Life and Illicit Love in Earlier Generations: Essays in Historical Sociology*. Cambridge, Cambridge University Press.

Lasch, C. (1975). *Haven in a Heartless World: The Family Besieged*. New York, Basic Books.

Lebovici, S. (1983). *Le Nourisson, la mère et le psychanalyste. Les interactions précoces*. Paris, Paidos le Centurion.

Le Coultre, R. (1972). *Psychoanalytische thema's en variaties* [Psychoanalytic themes and variations]. Deventer, Van Loghum Slaterus.

Lerner, H. E. (1976). 'Parental mislabeling of female genitals as a determinant of penis envy and learning inhibitions in women'. *Journal of the American Psycho-Analytic Association, Supplement Female Psychology*, 24, 269–283.

Le Roy Ladurie, E. (1984). *Montaillou: Village occitan de 1294 à 1324*. Paris, Gallimard.

Loftus, E. F. (1993). 'The reality of repressed memories'. *American Psychologist* 48, 518–537.

MacFarlane, A. (1978). *The Origins of English Individualism*. Oxford, Basil Blackwell.

Mahler, M. S. (1968). *On Human Symbiosis and the Vicissitudes of Individuation*. New York, International Universities Press.

Mahler, M. S. (1981). 'Aggression in the service of separation–individuation: Case study of a mother–daughter relationship'. *Psychoanalytic Quarterly*, 50, 625–638.

Mahler, M. S., Pine, F., & Bergman, A. (1975). *The Psychological Birth of the Human Infant: Symbiosis and Individuation*. London, Hutchinson.

Masson, J. M. (1984). *The Assault on Truth: Freud's Suppression of the Seduction Theory*. New York, Farrar, Straus & Giroux.

Masson, J. M. (Ed.) (1985). *The Complete Letters of Sigmund Freud to Wilhelm Fliess, 1887–1904*. Cambridge, MA/London, The Belknap Press of Harvard University Press.

McDougall, J. (1986). 'Eve's reflection: On the homosexual components of female sexuality', in H. C. Meyers (Ed.), *Between Analyst and Patient: New Dimensions in Countertransference and Transference*. Hillsdale, NJ, The Analytic Press, pp. 213–228.

McDougall, J. (1995). *The Many Faces of Eros: A Psychoanalytic Exploration of Human Sexuality*. New York/London, Norton.

Meissner, W. W. (2005). 'Gender identity and the self: II. Femininity, homosexuality, and the theory of the self'. *Psychoanalytic Review*, 92, 29–66.

Mentzos, S. (1993). *Hysterie: Zur Psychodynamik unbewuzster Inszenierungen*. Frankfurt am Main, Fischer Verlag.

Meyers, H. (1989). 'The impact of teenage children on parents', in J. M. Oldham & R. S. Liebert (Eds.), *The Middle Years: New Psychoanalytic Perspectives*. New Haven/London, Yale University Press, pp. 75–88.

Miller, A. (1981). *Du sollst nicht merken*. Frankfurt am Main, Suhrkamp.

Mitscherlich, A. (1992). *Society without the Father: A Contribution to Social Psychology*. Kindle Edition.

Modell, A. H. (1989). 'Object relations theory: Psychic aliveness in the middle years', in J. M. Oldham & R. S. Liebert (Eds.), *The Middle Years: New Psychoanalytic Perspectives*. New Haven/London, Yale University Press, pp. 17–26.

Mozart, W. A. (1948). *Briefe*. Zurich, Willi Reich, Menasse.

Munder Ross, J. (1990). 'The eye of the beholder: The developmental dialogue between fathers and daughters', in Robert A. Nemiroff & Calvin A. Colarusso (Eds.), *New Dimensions in Adult Development*. New York, Basic Books, 47–72.

Nagera, H. (1966). *Early Childhood Disturbances, the Infantile Neurosis, and the Adulthood Disturbances*. New York, International Universities Press.

Nemiroff, R. A., & Colarusso, C. A. (1981). *Adult Development: A New Dimension in Psychodynamic Theory and Practice*. New York/London, Plenum Press.

Nemiroff, R. A., & Colarusso, C. A. (1990). *New Dimensions in Adult Development*. New York, Basic Books.

Némirovski, I. (2006). *Suite Francaise*, tr. Sandra Smith. New York, Knopf.

Oldham, J. (1989). 'The third individuation: Middle-aged children and their parents', in J. M. Oldham & R. S. Liebert (Eds.), *The Middle Years: New Psychoanalytic Perspectives*. New Haven/London, Yale University Press, pp. 89–104.

Oliner, M. M. (1982). 'The anal phase', in D. Mendell (Ed.), *Early Female Development: Current Psychoanalytic Views*. Lancaster, MTP Press, pp. 24–59.

O'Neill, E. (1984 [1932]). *Mourning Becomes Electra*. London, Jonathan Cape.

Origo, I. (1963). *The Merchant of Prato: Daily Life in a Medieval Italian City*. Harmondsworth, UK, Penguin.

Ornstein, P. (1989). 'Self psychology: The fate of the nuclear self in the middle years', in J. M. Oldham & R. S. Liebert (Eds.), *The Middle Years: New Psychoanalytic Perspectives*. New Haven/London, Yale University Press, pp. 27–39.

Parens, H. (1990). 'On the girl's psychosexual development: Reconsiderations suggested from direct observation'. *Journal of the American Psycho-Analytic Association* 38, 743–772.

Pines, D. (1993). *A Woman's Unconscious Use of Her Body*. London, Virago.

Pitt, B. (1982). 'Depression and childbirth', in E. S. Paykel (Ed.), *Handbook of Affective Disorders*. Edinburgh, Churchill Livingstone, pp. 361–378.

Pollock, G. H. (1981). 'Aging or aged: Development or pathology', in S. I. Greenspan & G. H. Pollock (Eds.), *The Course of Life*. Madison, CT, International Universities Press.

Rangell, L. (1959). 'The nature of conversion'. *Journal of the American Psycho-Analytic Association* 7, 632–662.

Reich, W. (1961 [1948]). *Character Analysis*. New York, The Noonday Press, Farrar, Straus & Cudahy.

Richier, P., & Alexandre-Bidon, D. (1994). *L'enfance au moyen âge*. Paris, Seuil.

Riesman, D. (1950). *The Lonely Crowd*. New Haven, Yale University Press.

Roiphe, H., & Galenson, E. (1981). *Infantile Origins of Sexual Identity*. New York, International Universities Press.

Rotter, L. (1934). 'Zur Psychologie der weiblichen Sexualität'. *Internationale Zeitschrift für Psychoanalyse* 20, 367–374.

Rougemont, D. de (1939). *L'amour et l'occident*. Paris, Plon.

Rubin, L. (1979). *Women of a Certain Age: The Midlife Search for Self*. New York, Harper & Row.

Sarnoff, C. (1976). *Latency*. New York, Jason Aronson.

Schama, S. (1987). *The Embarrassment of Riches: An Interpretation of Dutch Culture in the Golden Age*. London, Fontana Press.

Schatzman, M. (1973). *Soul Murder: Persecution in the Family*. London, Penguin.

Schwartz, A. (1986). 'Some notes on the development of female gender role identity', in J. L. Alpert (Ed.), *Psychoanalysis and Women: Contemporary Reappraisals*. Hillsdale, NJ, The Analytic Press, pp. 57–82.

Shapiro, D. (1965). *Neurotic Styles*. New York, Basic Books.

Sheehy, G. (1976). *Silent Passages*. Houston/New York, Random House.

Shopper, M. (1979). 'The rediscovery of the vagina and the importance of the menstrual tampon', in M. Sugar (Ed.), *Female Adolescent Development*. New York, Brunner/Mazel, pp. 214–233.

Shorter, E. (1992). *From Paralysis to Fatigue: a History of Psychosomatic Illness in the Modern Era*. New York, Simon & Schuster.

Shorter, E. (1975). *The Making of the Modern Family*, Glasgow, Fontana Collins.

Showalter, E. (1997). *Hystories: Hysterical Epidemics and Modern Culture*. New York/ London, Columbia University Press/Picador.

Silverman, D. K. (1987). 'Female bonding: Some supportive findings for Melanie Klein's views'. *Psychoanalytic Review* 74, 201–215.

Simon, B. (1991). 'Is the Oedipus complex still the cornerstone of psychoanalysis?' *Journal of the American Psycho-Analytic Association* 39, 641–668.

Simon, B. (1992). ' "Incest – see under Oedipus complex". The history of an error in psychoanalysis'. *Journal of the American Psycho-Analytic Association* 40, 955–988.

Simon, B, & Blass, R. (1991). 'Developments and vicissitudes of Freud's ideas on the Oedipus complex', in J. Neu (Ed.), *The Cambridge Companion to Freud*. Cambridge, Cambridge University Press, pp. 161–174.

Sophocles (1953). *Electra and Other Plays*, tr. E. F. Watling. Harmondsworth, UK, Viking/Penguin.

Spitz, R. (1945). 'Hospitalism: An inquiry into the genesis of psychiatric conditions in early childhood'. *Psychoanalytic Study of the Child* 1, 53–74.

Stekel, W. (1908). *Nervöse Angstzustände und ihre Behandlung*. Berlin/Vienna, Verlag Urban & Schwarzenberg.

Stern, D. N. (1985). *The Interpersonal World of the Infant: A View from Psychoanalysis and Developmental Psychology*. New York, Basic Books.

Stern, D. N. (1995). *The Motherhood Constellation: A Unified View of Parent–Infant Psychotherapy*. Basic Books. New York.

Stoller, R. (1976). 'Primary femininity'. *Journal of the American Psycho-Analytic Association, Supplement: Female Sexuality*, 24, 59–78.

Stone, L. (1977). *The Family, Sex and Marriage in England 1500–1800*. London, Penguin.

Storr, A. (1995). 'The myth of repressed memory: False memories and allegations of sexual abuse'. *International Herald Tribune*, 23 January, 7.

Torok, M. (1970) [1964]). 'The significance of penis envy in women', in J. Chasseguet-Smirgel (Ed.), *Female Sexuality*. London, Maresfield, pp. 135–170.

Tyson, R. L., & Tyson, P. (1990). *Psychoanalytic Theories of Development and Integration*. New Haven/London, Yale University Press.

Ussel, J. M. W. van (1982). *De geschiedenis van het sexuele problem* [The history of the sexual problem]. Meppel, Boom.

Vaillant, G. E. (1989). 'The evolution of defense mechanisms during the middle years', in J. M. Oldham & R. S. Liebert (Eds.), *The Middle Years: New Psychoanalytic Perspectives*. New Haven/London, Yale University Press, pp. 58–72.

Van Haute, P. (2005). 'Infantile sexuality, primary object-love and the anthropological significance of the Oedipus complex: Re-reading Freud's "Female sexuality" '. *International Journal of Psycho-Analysis*, 86, 1661–1678.

Veith, I. (1965). *The History of Disease*. Chicago, The University of Chicago Press.

Verdoorn, Y. A. (1965). *Volksgezondheid en sociale ontwikkeling. Beschouwingen over het gezondheidswezen te Amsterdam in de 19e eeuw* [Public health and social development. Observations on healthcare in Amsterdam in the nineteenth century]. Utrecht, Aula Spectrum.

Viederman, M. (1989). 'Middle life as a period of mutative change', in J. M. Oldham & R. S. Liebert (Eds.), *The Middle Years: New Psychoanalytic Perspectives*. New Haven/London, Yale University Press, pp. 224–239.

Wagner, R. (1995). *Siegfried*. Stuttgart, Reclam.

Welldon, E. V. (1989). *Mother, Madonna, Whore: The Idealization and Denigration of Motherhood*. London, Heinemann.

Wind, E. de (1984). 'Some implications of former massive traumatization upon the actual analytic process'. *International Journal of Psycho-Analysis* 65, 273–281.

Winnicott, D. W. (1958). *Collected Papers*. London, Tavistock.

Winnicott, D. W. (1965). *The Family and Individual Development*. London, Tavistock.

Winnicott, D. W. (1972). *The Maturational Process and the Facilitating Environment*. London, The Hogarth Press.

Wisdom, J. O. (1961). 'A methodological approach to the problem of hysteria'. *International Journal of Psycho-Analysis* 42, 224–237.

Woolf, V. (1970) [1928]). *A Room of One's Own*. Harmondsworth, UK, Penguin.

Wright, N. (1988). *Mrs. Klein*. London, Walker Books.

Young-Bruehl, E. (1988). *Anna Freud*. London, Macmillan.

Young-Bruehl, E. (1989). 'Looking for Anna Freud's mother'. *Psychoanalytic Study of the Child* 44, 391–408.

Young-Bruehl, E. (Ed.) (1990). *Freud on Women*. New York/London, Norton & Company.

Zetzel, E. (1968). 'Contribution to a symposium on indications and contra-indications for psychoanalytic treatment: The so-called good hysteric'. *International Journal of Psycho-Analysis* 49, 256–260.

Index